EMERGENCY INFORMATION

My Veterinarian's name: _____, D.V.M.

Phone: _____

Hospital address: _____

Hospital phone: _____

Veterinary Society emergency phone: _____

Emergency Clinic address: _____

Area Poison-Control Center phone: _____

For Help with Wild or Stray Animals, phone:

    ASPCA: _____   Sheriff: _____

    Game Warden: _____   Police: _____

    Other: _____

For advice about animal bites to humans,
    Public-Health Officer phone: _____

My full-grown pet weighs: _____ Birthdate: _____

Its normal temperature: ____ pulse: ____ respirations: ____

First aid techniques for specific problems are indexed in bold type. Look there first!

First Aid for Pets

First Aid
for
Pets

Robert W. Kirk, D.V.M.

A Sunrise Book

E. P. DUTTON | NEW YORK

Grateful acknowledgment is made to the following for permission to use copyrighted materials: *Borden, Inc.* "Composition of Animal Milks" and "Substitutes for Maternal Milk" from *Pet-Vet Products.* Reprinted by permission of Borden, Inc./*Francis A. Kallfelz.* "Estimated Nutrient Requirements of Dogs and Cats" and "Energy and Protein Requirements of Growing Dogs and Cats" from *Current Veterinary Therapy V,* by R. W. Kirk. Copyright © 1974 by W. B. Saunders Co., Philadelphia. Reprinted by permission of the author./*Gary D. Osweiler, D.V.M.* "Some Chemical Products Hazardous to Pets" from *Current Veterinary Therapy VI,* by R. W. Kirk, D.V.M. Copyright © 1977 by W. B. Saunders Co., Philadelphia. Reprinted by permission of the author./*Stephen M. Schuchman, D.V.M.* "Useful Information" modified from "Individual Care and Treatment of Rabbits, Mice, Rats, Guinea Pigs, Hamsters and Gerbils" from *Current Veterinary Therapy VI,* by R. W. Kirk. Copyright © 1977 by W. B. Saunders Co., Philadelphia. Reprinted by permission of the author.

Library of Congress Cataloging in Publication Data
Kirk, Robert Warren, 1922–
First aid for pets.
"A Sunrise book."
Bibliography: p.
1. Pets—Diseases.   2. First aid for animals.
I. Title.
SF981.K5   1978   636.089′8′8   77-6309
ISBN: 0-87690-265-4 (cloth)
0-87690-275-1 (paper)
Published simultaneously in Canada by Clarke, Irwin & Company Limited, Toronto and Vancouver

Drawings by George Batik

Designed by Ann Gold

Notice

The first aid suggestions in this book are generalizations of safe and conservative methods for handling emergencies and other problems. Since each illness, injury, or other condition is a highly individual matter, subject to individual complications, *it is imperative that you seek and follow your own veterinarian's advice as soon as possible.*

Contents

II. First Aid Techniques

III. Miscellaneous Problem Solving

Appendixes

How to Use This Book

This book is meant to be a pet first aid manual—and more. It is written for the concerned pet owner, to provide simple, safe, and effective veterinary advice for many animal emergencies. The text is primarily concerned with the veterinary problems of dogs and cats, but some attention is directed to birds and other small pets. Although the text places major emphasis on temporary measures for handling *emergency* situations—many of them life threatening—there is considerable discussion about a variety of *common,* but troublesome problems as well.

There is just too much material to be assimilated when you find your pet in need of first aid. The expanded information this book contains will give you a better understanding of your pet and the predicaments that may arise.

To use this information intelligently, you should

1. Know your pet well, so you can recognize the unusual behavior that is a sign of illness.

2. Read the book from cover to cover, to strengthen your knowledge about potential problems and methods of dealing with them.

3. Learn the first aid techniques, such as restraint, bandaging, and administering medication, described in Part II.

4. Practice on your own pet so you both will be familiar with procedures that may be life saving in an emergency, and your pet will more readily accept them.

5. Record the data requested in the outline on the first page

now! This is your panic pacifier, and it will give you fingertip sources of help when they are urgently needed.

6. Prepare a first aid kit, such as the one described on page 145 *now!* Learn the indications for each of its components and discuss their use with your veterinarian. Be prepared!

7. Choose your veterinarian carefully; trust him and know him. Allow him to know you, so that when you call in an emergency, he can visualize your problem and understand your explanation of the situation.

Understanding the basic principles and procedures of preventive medicine will help you to safeguard your pet from possible injuries and will enable you to deal effectively with emergencies should they arise.

The information in this book is derived from more than thirty years of active experience with small animals and complemented by the ideas and knowledge of innumerable professional colleagues, whose thoughts and methods I have assimilated over the years.

The line drawings are the work of George Batik, and the photographs are by John Lauber; both men are members of the Biomedical Communications Section, New York State College of Veterinary Medicine, Cornell University.

My wife, Helen, a registered nurse, has been a partner in the production and clarification of the ideas presented here, as she has in everything I have done.

All those who have worked to organize the information in this book hope the emergency care will never be needed for your pet. If it is, we are confident our suggestions will help you to alleviate suffering, prevent further injury—and even save a life.

ROBERT W. KIRK, D.V.M.

Ithaca, New York
April 1977

I.

FIRST AID FOR ACCIDENTS AND ILLNESS

1.

What Is First Aid?

Definition and Objectives

First aid is the immediate care given an animal that is suffering from the effects of an accident or sudden illness. First aid also covers the initial treatment of diseases that have "just been discovered" by the owner but that have in reality been present for some time.

When we administer first aid to an animal, we are handicapped by the patient's inability to communicate verbally; we may have difficulty telling when, how, or where an injury occurred or an illness started. Fortunately, with experience, we can learn to "read" an animal's reactions, which convey a great deal of information. But we still cannot explain our motives to the injured patient when applying first aid.

An injured animal will be frightened and in pain—and thus uncooperative. It will usually attempt to run away and hide (especially a cat) and must often be captured and forcibly restrained (see pages 151–165). We may be bitten, scratched, or otherwise harmed by the frantic patient. Our use of muzzles, blankets, bags, and other protective measures, together with firm but gentle handling, often "tells" the patient that we are in control but compassionate. Talking quietly to the animal and using its name frequently often has a calming and reassuring effect.

Knowledge of successful methods of handling animals, as well as a recognition of normal structures and functions of the animal body, is a great help in understanding and dealing with problems as they arise.

The key objectives of first aid are:
1. To preserve life.
2. To alleviate suffering.
3. To promote recovery.
4. To prevent aggravation of the injury or illness until we can obtain veterinary assistance.

FIRST AID PROCEDURES IN LIFE-THREATENING EMERGENCIES

1. *Remove the cause* of the injury if possible.

2. *Clear airways* so the animal can breathe. Remove collar and any foreign material, blood, or fluids from the nose and throat (see pages 14 and 70–72). Place the animal in the position that makes breathing as easy as possible.

3. *Give artificial respiration* if the patient is not breathing (see pages 14–16).

4. *Treat cardiac arrest* immediately. Often a sharp blow on the side of the chest, just behind the shoulder, will suffice. Repeat every 15 seconds until patient responds. Failure after 5 minutes of effort means the patient has died.

5. *Stop or control bleeding* as soon as possible. Use pressure bandages, pressure points, or tourniquets as needed (see pages 23–28).

6. *Cover any wounds* with clean, dry dressings (see pages 167–176).

7. *Keep the patient warm* (blankets, box, warm car).

8. *Do not move* or manipulate the patient unnecessarily. An injured animal will usually assume the least painful position, with the injured part uppermost. When it is necessary to move the patient, support and protect the injured area to prevent further

damage and pain. Use blankets, rugs, and boards or boxes to support an animal being transported. (See pages 148–149.)

9. *Treat for shock* (see pages 37–42). If the animal is unconscious, place its head slightly lower than the rest of its body to treat shock and to prevent the patient from inhaling fluids or materials in the mouth. *Do not give anything by mouth.* If the animal is conscious and not seriously injured, you may give small amounts of drinking water.

10. *Promptly transport the animal to a veterinary facility* for professional care.

11. If possible, *have someone phone the veterinary hospital* (while you are on your way) to alert the staff of your need for emergency care. The person who calls should give a brief description of the injuries, so the hospital personnel can make preparations for your arrival.

12. *Don't speed* on the way! A patient that won't survive a few minutes probably can't be saved—and the rough ride to the hospital may aggravate injuries. Risking an additional accident is not justified by any emergency.

2.

Responsibility and Planning to Prevent Accidents and Illness

Selecting and Keeping a Pet

Carefully considered selection of your pet can prevent many problems that would require first aid.

That happy little ball of squirming love may be irresistible at the time you first see it. However, when it has, within a year, matured to 160 pounds and begun to sweep priceless art objects from the coffee table with its wagging tail, your love may evaporate. *Don't be an impulse buyer.*

One should really *want* a pet. Having made this decision, determine what needs a pet will fulfill for you and what it will require of you for its own happiness and health.

Housing and husbandry (management) needs should be considered first. In oriental countries and crowded apartment complexes, where space is a crucial factor, crickets, mice, birds, and fish are popular pets. These are especially good for shut-ins. In quarters that provide more space, cats and dogs are sensible choices, while in country or suburban areas even horses can be kept comfortably.

Exotic species of birds, cats, monkeys, and other wild animals are occasionally kept as pets but they have serious drawbacks for the average individual. Not only do they often need special housing and food, but they may transmit diseases to man and can be physically dangerous. You should really do some soul-searching and get expert advice before selecting a pet from this group of animals.

Once you have selected the species, you can get down to selecting a breed with the characteristics that you want. Dogs, for instance, come in all sizes and temperaments, with a variety of hair coat and thus of grooming needs. Some are suitable for families with children, others for guard duties. Some do well in confined living quarters; others have a special need for exercise. In city areas the disposal of voluminous bowel movements can be a major problem and should be a deterrent to selecting a large breed. Many breeds are easily trained, but there are some that have a tendency to fight or are headstrong and hard to control. One of the advantages of purebred animals over mongrels is the general predictability of the purebred's mature characteristics. Most mongrels make excellent pets, however.

Breed and sex may have a real influence on the future health problems of your pet. The inconvenience of animals "in season" or of having young can be avoided by buying a male or having a female neutered—a responsibility of utmost importance these days because of the overpopulation of stray dogs. Male dogs and cats tend to be bold and outgoing, while spayed (neutered) females tend to be more placid and have closer ties and affection for the home. Incidentally, with proper feeding, there is no reason why a spayed female should become obese.

The breed you select may have a high incidence of specific health problems, such as eye, ear, or skin disease. However, other breeds "age early," have joint or bone problems, allergies, neuroses, or infirmities you may wish to avoid. A veterinarian can give helpful advice about the medical problems you may encounter in certain breeds and can often help you choose a breed with the general traits that best fit your needs. Contact the American Kennel Club, 51 Madison Avenue, New York, N.Y. 10010, for additional information.

Training and proper socialization (teaching the pet its proper place in animal and human society) are vital to having a happy animal that fits into your environment and is a pleasure to have around. One of the best reasons for buying a puppy at 7 weeks of age is to allow you the opportunity to properly train it. If you purchase a puppy at an older age, many of its habits will already be firmly established. If they are good habits, you are lucky. If they are bad ones, you could have a real problem. Training a dog to obey your commands—especially to come, to stay with you, to stay on your property, and to avoid traffic—is important in preventing injury from accidents, fights, or poisoning. Dog obedience classes, which train you to train your dog, are excellent. Alternatively, professional trainers may be useful in making your dog a good citizen.

The comments above have referred primarily to dogs, but cats may make better pets for some people. They are independent and almost impossible to train to your will. Fortunately, they train themselves in many important ways. They adapt well to apartments, need little exercise, and usually housebreak themselves if a litter box is provided. On the other hand, they often fight with other cats if they are allowed to wander. They may be injured by automobiles, by falls out of windows or trees, or by marauding dogs. Cats are easily poisoned as a result of fastidious habits in cleaning their hair coats.

Coat type should be a further consideration in selecting your pet. The hair coat of your dog or cat is a mirror that reflects your pet's general health. You must provide the needed grooming. Short coats can be quickly brushed and need shampooing infrequently. Long coats may need daily combing and frequent bathing or periodic trips to the groomer for trimming or plucking. It takes time and costs money to keep your pet looking its best, but this care is essential for keeping the animal's skin healthy and free of parasites. If you haven't time to devote to the care a long coat requires, you should get a short-coated pet.

Vaccinations are extremely effective in preventing infectious diseases of dogs and cats. Immunizations prevent many contagious diseases from spreading among dogs and cats, but regular booster injections are needed to maintain the best protection. Rabies vaccination not only protects your pet but is an essential public health measure. A person or pet bitten by a rabid animal may contract this fatal disease. Cooperate with your veterinarian in planning a total health-care plan for your pet. Prevention is better than first aid!

Vaccines (see pages 227–229) provide excellent protection for the following diseases:

Dogs	*Cats*
Distemper	Panleukopenia (feline distemper)
Hepatitis	Respiratory infections
Leptospirosis	Rabies
Rabies	

Infectious bronchitis (kennel cough)
Tetanus (for dogs that are housed with horses)

Shipping Pets

Shipping pets by air is usually safe, but it does require planning ahead and attention to details.

1. Make reservations with the airline well in advance. It is best to avoid weekend travel if possible.

2. Determine which vaccinations, health certificates, and other papers are needed for shipment. The airlines will tell you. These requirements vary with the destination and are especially important for pets traveling to foreign countries. Some places allow pets to enter only after they are held in quarantine for many months (England, Australia, Hawaii).

Make arrangements to have the necessary papers in plenty of time before departure. Tranquilization for the trip may be desirable in certain cases. Discuss this with your veterinarian when you get the health certificate(s) for the trip.

3. Purchase an approved shipping kennel from the airlines or your pet store. It must have a solid, waterproof bottom and ventilation openings on at least two sides. No openings near the bottom should be large enough to allow your pet's foot to be caught outside. The kennel must be sturdy, escape-proof, and light in weight. A crate made of fiberglass or plywood is suitable. The dimensions depend on your pet's height at the shoulder.

a. For shoulder heights up to 15 inches (cats, beagles, poodles, small terriers) a kennel 26″ x 18″ x 19″ high is adequate.
b. For shoulder heights up to 22 inches (spaniels, Dalmations, bassets, corgis, large terriers) a kennel 36″ x 22″ x 26″ high is adequate.
c. For shoulder heights up to 25 inches (collies, Dobermans, retrievers, setters) a kennel 43″ x 25″ x 30″ high is adequate.
d. For giant breeds, special kennels may be needed.

4. Your pet may accept the kennel as "home" better if it is housed in the kennel for several nights before the trip. Having slept there, the animal will probably feel more secure on the trip because it is in a familiar place.

5. Feed your pet lightly for 2 days before traveling and give it a small meal 6 to 8 hours before flight time. Do not allow excessive water. Exercise the animal several times before flight time to allow for bladder and bowel evacuations.

6. If travel time will be less than 24 hours, provide a small amount of water in the kennel container—but no food. If travel time will be longer, attach a small cloth bag containing dry or semi-moist food to the outside of the kennel and provide brief feeding directions.

7. Place shredded paper in the bottom of the kennel and put the traveling pet into the kennel just before flight time. Plan to arrive at the airport at least one hour before departure for check-in at the appropriate air freight or passenger terminal. A pet traveling with you, as "excess baggage," may have a faster and better flight than a pet that flies air freight.

8. Make arrangements for prompt pick-up or delivery at your destination. Label the kennel and shipping documents with the appropriate telephone contacts in case problems develop during the trip.

9. If you are shipping by air freight, telephone the person receiving the pet and tell him the flight number, the actual time of

departure, the scheduled time of arrival, and any other details you feel are important. If things do become disorganized, someone can start checking immediately.

10. Relax. Your pet will be clean and comfortable, since it will be traveling in the same environment as the passengers.

3.

Emergency
Respiratory Problems

Definition

A respiratory emergency is any condition that causes breathing to stop or that reduces oxygen intake to a low level, thus threatening life.

Artificial respiration is a first aid technique that causes air to flow into and out of the lungs (so oxygen can be carried to the heart and brain) of a patient that is not breathing adequately.

Causes

1. Obstruction of the pharynx or air passages. This may be caused by a foreign body such as a bone, chunk of food, or wood; by fluids (mucus, vomited matter, or blood from injuries); by swelling from burns, corrosive poisons, or severe injuries by tight collars; or by spasms of the larynx or asthma. The tongue may also swell or fall back into the throat and add to the obstruction.

2. Asphyxia by depletion of oxygen in the air or replacement of oxygen by toxic gases or smoke. Animals trapped in old refrigerators, small boxes, cisterns or wells, silos, sewers, barrels, or areas with carbon monoxide or escaping toxic gases will be deprived of enough oxygen to support life and may die within a few minutes. Always dispose of plastic bags promptly and properly. Pets may become tangled in them and suffocate.

Some gases are explosive (e.g., cooking, heating, and mine gas), and fire, electric switches, or static electricity may trigger an explosion, adding this hazard to that of asphyxia.

  3. Miscellaneous factors

    a. Strangulation by an accidentally snagged collar (see page 17).

    b. Smoke inhalation (see pages 56–57).

    c. Electrocution (see pages 75–76 and 150).

    d. Drowning (see page 17).

    e. Poisoning that depresses respiration or weakens breathing muscles as part of its toxic effect.

    f. Chest injuries. Crushing wounds may damage the lungs; puncture wounds, fractured ribs, and other severe injuries may let air into the chest and so destroy the normal bellows action of the lungs. This condition is called pneumothorax. Even though the animal tries, it cannot inhale and exhale adequate amounts of air.

      Crushing chest injuries are commonly caused by entanglement with machinery, automobile accidents, severe falls, and kicks from horses or other large animals. Chest wounds may also be associated with these incidents, but gunshot or arrow wounds, deep lacerations or stabs from glass, spikes, other sharp instruments, or even sticks may produce serious lesions. (See also pages 22–23 and 84–86.)

Signs and Symptoms

  1. The animal's lips, tongue, and inner eyelids may be dark red or bluish in color.

  2. Respirations may stop, be slow and shallow, or gasping. The patient may sit down but extend its neck, elevate its nose, open its mouth, and gasp to try to breathe more easily.

  3. The patient may be unconscious.

  4. The pupils of the eye may become dilated after a few minutes of respiratory arrest—an ominous sign.

FIRST AID FOR
RESPIRATORY EMERGENCIES:
ARTIFICIAL RESPIRATION

PRINCIPLES

1. Clear and maintain an open airway from the nose and mouth to the lungs.

2. Restore or assist breathing, so that adequate air flows in and out of the lungs. This is usually provided by artificial respiration.

PROCEDURES

1. Open the animal's mouth, grasp the tongue with cloth or paper so it won't slip, and pull it well forward. Keep it there and examine the back of the mouth for obstructions. Remove them by swabbing with Q-tips or gauze or cloth sponges, or by hooking a foreign body with your fingers (see pages 68–71).

2. Remove any collar, rope, or constricting item.

3. If the animal has fluid in its throat or is a drowning victim, grasp the rear legs and hold the animal upside down for 15 to 30 seconds. If the patient is large, place it on a sloping surface, with the head lower than the chest and the rest of the body. This facilitates drainage of fluids from the lungs.

4. Begin artificial respiration at once (see Figure 1). Place the animal on its sioe on a firm surface. Extend the head and neck and pull the tongue forward. Place both hands on the ribs immediately behind the animal's shoulder blade. With your hands give a sudden downward thrust. This compresses the animal's chest and expels the air from the lungs. Release the hand pressure immediately. The elasticity of the chest causes it to expand so the lungs fill with air. Repeat this procedure at a rate of about 12 times per minute.

If the chest cavity has been punctured or has an open wound connecting the inside of the chest to outside air, the above method

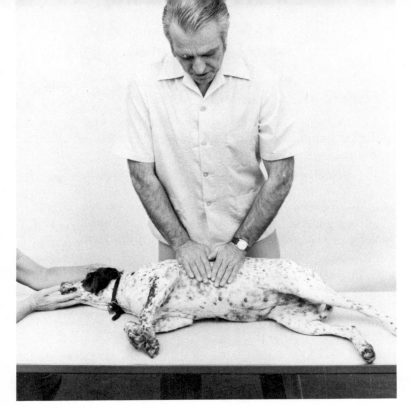

FIGURE 1. *Artificial respiration*. Place the patient on its side on a firm surface and extend the head and neck (in a straight line with the spine). Pull the tongue forward. Place both hands on the side of the chest near the last rib and press down firmly 12 times per minute. Release quickly and completely at the end of each compression.

will not be effective. Hold the patient's mouth and lips closed, place your mouth tightly over the animal's nose, and blow firmly into its nostrils. The air pressure will expand the animal's lungs from the inside to provide the necessary air exchange to maintain life. Blow for 3 seconds, relax for 2 seconds, and repeat.

In the above case, close the wound and pad it with bandages or clean cloths taped firmly in place to seal the wound (see pages 23 and 85). Transport the patient quickly to a veterinary hospital for proper care, continuing the resuscitative measures on the way.

Chest injuries as described here are often fatal without immediate first aid measures and professional care.

5. Continue artificial respiration until the patient is breathing by itself or is pronounced dead. Often 30 to 60 minutes' effort will be necessary.

6. Cardiac arrest may occur soon after respiratory arrest. The animal is in cardiac arrest if you cannot feel the heartbeat at the lower part of the chest just behind the patient's left elbow or by taking the pulse (see pages 189–191 and figures 2 and 48, page 190). If this occurs, strike the chest sharply with your fist once or twice in the region just behind the shoulder. Cardiac massage offers little hope unless a team of trained first-aiders is available on the spot.

FIGURE 2. *The apex heartbeat.* Count the heartbeat by feeling the left side of the patient's chest, just behind the elbow.

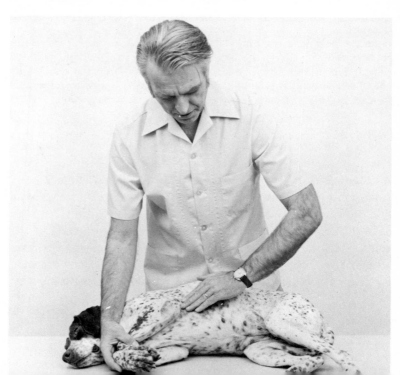

Prevention

1. Obstruction. Provide as playthings (balls, bones, and toys) only items that are too large to be swallowed by your pet or to become lodged in its throat.

2. Asphyxia. Permanently remove latches from abandoned refrigerators and freezers. Be aware that the lack of ventilation in boxes, barrels, closets, or other small rooms can also be hazardous to your pet. Do not shut the damper of the fireplace until the fire is completely out. Remember that the gases from a closed-in, dying fire can be deadly. At any sign of gas odors or other "funny" smell, notify your public utility repair service—open windows and doors and get out of the building with your pet until the service representatives arrive.

3. Strangulation. A hunting dog may get its collar snagged and choke as it struggles to get free. Provide a "breakaway" or stretch collar. Never tie a dog to a fence that it can jump over, too near a stairway, or close to a steep bank. If it climbs over the fence or falls down the stairs or bank, the animal may "hang" itself.

4. Drowning. Dogs and cats are naturally adequate swimmers and can negotiate short distances well. However, they are in danger of drowning if they are obliged to swim a long distance or if they should fall into a pool with steep sides that prevent them from climbing out. If you own a pool, provide a ramp exit (animals can't climb ladders) and teach your pet to use it.

5. Poisoning. Keep medicines and poisons stored where your pet does not have access to them.

4.

Allergic Reactions

Definition

An allergic reaction is the animal body's abnormal response to the invasion of a foreign substance—usually a protein material. The substance can be inhaled (pollens), ingested (spoiled meat or special foods), or injected (insect venom or certain drugs). The reaction is rarely a severe problem, since most are local or minor in nature. However, when difficult breathing or circulatory collapse develops, the problem can be an extreme emergency and can cause death.

Causes

The causative agent is usually something that the animal has encountered before, and the animal's reaction may become worse with each new exposure. Animals may develop local contact allergies to leather, metal, flea collars, certain weeds, plastic dishes, and nylon or wool rugs. They also develop local swelling and redness as the result of bites from such insects as wasps, bees, mosquitos, and fleas. In certain animals, a bee or wasp sting may produce a life-threatening generalized reaction (anaphylaxis) as well. Inhalation of plant pollens (ragweed, tree or grass pollens) or ingestion of spoiled meat or special foods (milk, seafood, or wheat) may also produce allergic reactions.

Types of Reactions

1. *Rapidly developing, or acute, allergic reactions* that cause collapse. The animal will become restless, will pant, drool, vomit, or have diarrhea, collapse, and even die. The patient may have a seizure (fit) during the acute stage. It may develop an asthmatic attack (constriction of the air passages).

This type of severe allergic reaction may develop from a drug injection, vaccine, insect sting, or ingestion of a special food.

2. *Slower developing allergic reactions* that cause hives. The animal develops soft raised swellings around the eyes, ears, and other areas of the face. These hives may itch, making the patient paw or rub the affected areas. Lesions appear after eating spoiled protein material or a special food or receiving an insect bite. They may also result from a blood transfusion, vaccine, or contact with certain chemicals. Inhalation of plant pollens rarely causes the hay-fever syndrome seen in man, but many dogs develop an itchy skin disease as a result of this type of allergy.

Response to first aid is usually good.

FIRST AID FOR
ACUTE ALLERGIC REACTIONS

1. Rapid treatment (injection of adrenalin) is necessary; so get veterinary help at once.

2. Ensure a clear airway. Give artificial respiration (see pages 14–16) if necessary—or oxygen if it's available.

FIRST AID FOR
HIVELIKE ALLERGIC REACTIONS

1. Watch for the onset of difficult breathing and get patient to a veterinary hospital quickly if it develops.

2. Wash the skin free of any known chemical residues.

3. Give a laxative of milk of magnesia (see pages 244 and 253 *and* an enema (see pages 194–196) if you think the patient has ingested a noxious substance.

4. Avoid reexposure to the causative agent.

5. Consult a veterinarian about the generalized skin reaction due to pollens. This usually occurs seasonally and requires professional diagnosis and desensitization treatments.

Prevention

The most effective prevention is to keep the pet from exposure to substances known to cause reactions. Desensitization injections may be helpful for certain kinds of pollen or inhalant allergies.

5.

Wounds and Bleeding

Definition

A wound is a break in the continuity of the body tissues. It may be internal, or it may be on the skin surface, penetrating to any depth.

Classification of Wounds

1. *An open wound* is an external break in the skin or mucous membranes.

2. *A closed wound* involves damaged internal tissues but there is no external break in the skin or mucous membranes.

Open Wounds

CAUSES

Forceful impact with external objects, such as in automobile accidents; stepping on sharp stones or pieces of glass or metal, bumping into wire fences or sharp sticks, or receiving blows from sharp tools or instruments.

Bite or claw wounds from fights with other animals are also frequent, but, fortunately, gunshot wounds and other injuries maliciously or accidentally inflicted by man and his tools or instruments are rare.

TYPES OF OPEN WOUNDS

There are five types of open wounds: abrasions, incisions, lacerations, punctures, and avulsions.

1. *Abrasions* are areas where the outer skin is damaged by scraping against a hard, rough surface. There is limited bleeding, although oozing of blood or serum is usually present. Gross contamination and infection are also usually present. Abrasions are painful. A hard crust forms over the damaged skin and healing takes place beneath its protective cover. In man, examples of abrasions are floor burns or scrapes from falling on a sidewalk. In animals, scrapes from contact with paved or gravel roads are common causes.

2. *Incisions* (cuts) are thin, cleanly made divisions of tissue produced by sharp instruments, broken glass, or sharp metal edges. These wounds often cause profuse bleeding. If they are deep, they may sever muscles, tendons, or nerves, as well as major blood vessels.

3. *Lacerations* are wounds that are irregular or jagged in outline, resulting from a great force that tears the soft tissues. Lacerations are deep, associated with extensive bleeding, and usually accompanied by gross contamination. This means healing will usually be complicated by infection. Bite wounds are common causes of lacerations.

4. *Punctures* are wounds produced by objects that pierce the skin, producing only a small hole on entry but (often) extensively damaging internal tissues and causing internal bleeding and deep contamination. The risk of infection in puncture wounds is increased because the bleeding is often minor and consequently there is limited "flushing action" of the blood to cleanse the wound. Puncture wounds can be caused by large thorns, splinters, needles, nails, or by stabbing with a knife or pitchfork.

5. *Avulsions* are wounds that result from the forcible separation of a mass of tissue from the animal's body. Extensive bleeding usually accompanies such injuries, and since a large amount of tissue is exposed, severe contamination can be expected. These

wounds usually accompany major accidents and body-crushing injuries. Explosions, dog fights, and gunshots are common causes of avulsions.

FIRST AID FOR OPEN WOUNDS

PRINCIPLES

1. Stop the bleeding first.

2. Protect the wound to prevent contamination.

3. Treat for shock if signs are present.

4. Seek veterinary care promptly.

FIRST AID FOR BLEEDING

PROCEDURES

1. Handle the patient gently but firmly—and carefully. Remember, an injured pet is afraid and in pain.

2. Muzzle the patient first. Restrain by holding the animal on its side or wrapping it in a blanket (see pages 151–152 and 157–164). Expose the injured part for treatment.

3. Cover the patient's eyes and speak calmly and quietly. It may be especially helpful to stroke the animal's head and repeat its name frequently. ("Good boy, Sport, good boy. It's okay, Sport.")

4. Act immediately! Rapid bleeding can cause shock and death in just a few minutes.

5. Stop the bleeding by

   a. *Applying direct pressure to the wound.* Place a sterile gauze pad or a clean handkerchief or cloth on the wound and apply firm, steady pressure over the entire wound

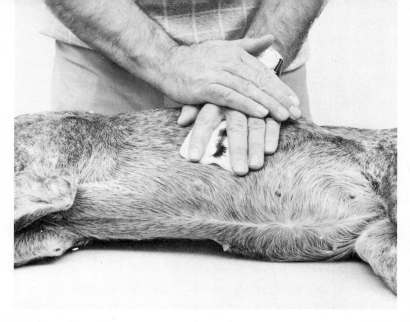

FIGURE 3. *Stopping bleeding.* Place a sterile gauze pad over the wound and apply firm pressure to stop bleeding.

surface with the palm of the hand (see Figure 3). The pad absorbs blood, allows clotting, and helps protect the wound from further contamination.

In most cases this method will stop the bleeding, especially if the wound is small and its edges can be pushed together as pressure is applied. For minor wounds, bandage the pad in place (see pages 167–174) and make arrangements to transport the patient to a veterinarian (see pages 148–149).

If blood soaks through the pad, add more padding and apply more pressure. Then bandage firmly in place. This is a pressure bandage (see figures 4 and 40, pages 25 and 175).

b. *Elevating the wound.* This method may be effective if the wound is on the leg and your pet is docile. However, elevation is less successful with animals than with people, since

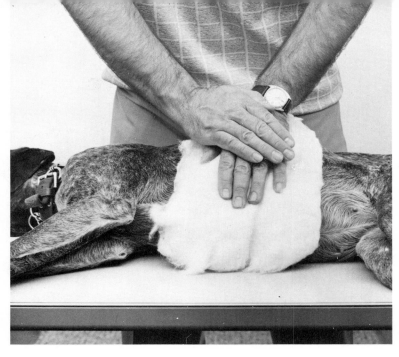

FIGURE 4. *A pressure bandage.* If bleeding continues, cover with cotton padding and apply more pressure. Add a many-tailed binder to maintain the pressure (see Figure 40, page 175).

animals are more restless and move around a lot more when they have been injured.

c. *Applying pressure to the artery* supplying the wounded area. If bleeding does not stop by direct pressure to the wound or by elevation, the "pressure point" technique may help. There are only three major pressure points in dogs and cats (see Figure 5, page 26). They are located at

    i. The upper inside of the front leg. Pressure here helps control bleeding of the lower forelimb by compressing the brachial artery.

    ii. The upper inside of the rear leg. Pressure here helps control bleeding of the lower hind limb by compressing the femoral artery.

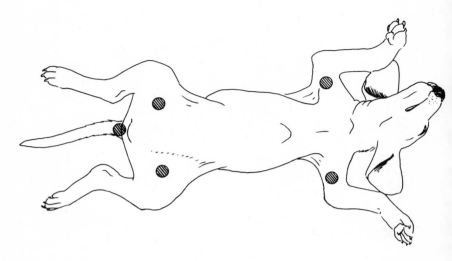

FIGURE 5. *The pressure points.* The major "pressure points" of dogs and cats are located at the shaded areas.

  iii. The underside of the tail near the point where it attaches to the body. Pressure here helps control bleeding of the tail by compressing the ventral coccygeal artery.

  Pressure may be applied in any of these areas. The objective is to compress the artery against the underlying bone. Always use the flat surface of the fingers, not the thumb or fingertips. At the same time continue to apply direct pressure to the wound. Release the pressure point after the bleeding is under control.

 d. *Applying a tourniquet* (see Figure 6). A tourniquet is a constricting band of cloth, gauze, or cord, wrapped around a limb to constrict blood vessels and control bleeding. This is a dangerous technique and should be used *only as a last resort, to save a life.* A tourniquet must be applied tightly to be effective; however, if it is left on for a long time, it will completely stop circulation to the dependent area and can cause the tissue to become gangrenous.

Once a tourniquet is applied, tighten it just enough to stop the bleeding and then leave it. Immediately transport the patient to a veterinary hospital.

FIGURE 6. *A tourniquet.* A tourniquet is applied to a dog's leg to control severe bleeding. Obtain a 2″ narrow strip of cloth. Wrap it twice around the leg and tie a half-hitch. Place a stick on top of the half hitch and then tie a square knot over the stick. Twist the stick gently until the bleeding slows. Secure the stick by tying a cloth strip around the stick and the patient's leg.

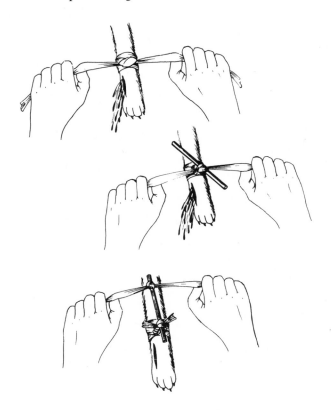

To apply a tourniquet

   i. Use a bandage or cloth strip 1 inch wide. (String or rope tends to cut tissues and produce more damage.)

   ii. Wrap twice around the leg or tail—*never* the neck! —to 2 inches from the wound, between the wound and the body. Tie a half hitch.

   iii. Place a pencil or stick on top of the half hitch and then tie a square knot above the stick.

   iv. Twist the stick gently until bleeding slows to a slight ooze.

   v. Secure the stick by tying with a bandage or wrapping a piece of tape around the stick and the leg or tail.

   vi. Cover the *wound surface* with sterile gauze or clean cloth. *Do not* cover the tourniquet.

   vii. Treat for shock (see pages 39–41).

   viii. Transport the patient to a veterinary hospital quickly.

6. *Prevent wound contamination.* All open wounds are contaminated unless they have been made in a sterile surgery. Measures to limit infection are generally associated with control of heavy bleeding. These wounds are usually covered with gauze or cloth pads and bandaged.

   a. Never put cotton batting directly on a wound.

   b. Never remove or disturb the original gauze cover. Let your veterinarian do it.

   c. Do not wash, cleanse, or probe the wound.

7. Treat for shock (see pages 39–41).

FIRST AID FOR OPEN WOUNDS THAT DO NOT NEED CONTROL OF BLEEDING

These are usually minor and can be treated by the first-aider.

1. Muzzle and restrain the patient (see pages 151–152 and 157–165).

2. Wash your hands and get your first aid kit (see page 145).

3. Clip the hair around the wound with a pair of scissors. Before you start, moisten or smear the hair with a thin film of ointment. This will make the hair stick together and to the scissors, so it won't get into the wound. As you cut, "fold" the hair away from the wound; this will also help keep the injured area clean.

4. Gently cleanse the wound with plain tap water and wash the skin around the wound with antiseptic soap and water.

5. Moisten a cotton-tipped applicator (Q-tip) and use it to wipe foreign material from the wound. Be very gentle, and do not probe deeply.

6. Blot the wound dry with sterile gauze (or even clean paper towels in an emergency).

7. Apply antiseptic or antibiotic wound medication.

8. Cover with a wound dressing (gauze pad) and bandage gently but firmly. Place several thicknesses of gauze, cloth, or cotton on top of the gauze wound dressing as padding before applying the bandage. (See pages 166–176 for dressing and bandaging directions.)

9. Replace the dressing and bandage every other day.

10. Get veterinary advice if you have questions or if signs of infection appear.

Wound Infections

All wounds have potential for infection, but if the contamination is minimal and the animal's natural defenses are normally active, they will successfully eliminate most bacterial infections and prevent any obvious symptoms of infection.

Dogs and cats are relatively resistant to tetanus; so in most cases you needn't be concerned about your pet's contracting this disease. There is an exception to this rule, however. Horse manure, horses, horse stalls, and implements used around stables may carry tetanus bacteria. Wounds sustained in this environment may need tetanus prophylaxis. Ask your veterinarian for guidance.

SIGNS AND SYMPTOMS

1. Pain, redness, and disuse of the affected part.
2. Swelling and local heat.
3. Pus draining from the wound or collected under crusts or bandages.
4. General body fever (over 103.5° F./40° C.).
5. General lethargy and decreased appetite.

FIRST AID FOR WOUND INFECTIONS

1. Remove bandages and gently lift off any crusts.

2. Prepare a soaking solution, using 2 teaspoons of salt to 1 pint hot (but not scalding) water.

3. Moisten a towel or cloth with this solution and place over the wound for 15 minutes every 2 hours. The towel should be comfortably hot to the touch.

4. Rinse the wound carefully with the above solution—or an alternate solution of 1 teaspoon of chlorine bleach in 1 quart of warm water.

5. Try to drain all pus away from the wound.

6. Apply antibiotic or other general antibacterial treatment. This is mandatory. Get the patient to a veterinarian promptly.

Special Wound Problems

1. Foreign objects may remain in wounds and cause infection and/or continuing damage. Thorns, slivers of wood, or glass fragments cause constant irritation and should be removed. If it is obvious, remove the foreign object with sterilized forceps, tweezers, or a needle. To sterilize the instrument, clean it carefully and hold it in a flame or soak it in alcohol.

2. Deeply imbedded larger objects, such as sticks, nails, or metal shafts may cause severe internal damage. Leave them in place for removal in the veterinary hospital. Before transporting a patient impaled by a foreign object, cut off the object near the skin surface and apply a large, padded bandage to the wound area; this will help immobilize the object and prevent further injury.

3. See pages 70–71 for removal of fishhooks, needles, etc.

4. Animal bites present complicated problems. Even a healthy mouth normally has a very large number of bacteria; this means that infection is probable. One must *always* be concerned that the bite may have been caused by a rabid animal.

Animal bites can produce punctures, lacerations, or avulsions. They are painful, since they do extensive soft-tissue damage to deep structures. Although perhaps only producing a puncture wound externally, a tooth may swing in a large arc under the victim's skin and sever muscles, tendons, and blood vessels. Because the bite is made through fur, hair is often pushed into the wound by the teeth. Thus, all bites must be thoroughly cleansed and protected with antibacterial dressings and anti-infection medication (see page 255). Cats, particularly, give and receive extremely painful bites that are prone to severe infection. Cats can inflict serious wounds with their sharp claws, too. An aroused cat is a formidable adversary; it usually defeats or escapes from all but the fiercest of dogs.

Rabies, or "hydrophobia," is a term that strikes fear in the heart of the pet owner, but that fear is usually exaggerated. Rabies is controlled well in pets that have been properly and regularly vaccinated. Wild creatures—especially skunks, foxes, and bats—are the common carriers of rabies; so bites from these animals are of major concern. Rabid wild creatures may act especially friendly or "strange" in comparison to their normal timidity. Try to avoid these wild animals, but if one bites your pet, you would be wise to kill the attacking animal and have it examined for rabies by public-health officials. If possible, avoid damaging the animal's head. Do not risk being bitten yourself by trying to capture it!

A pet with an up-to-date rabies vaccination is protected against rabies even if it is bitten by a rabid animal.

Keep rabies vaccinations current!

If your pet is bitten by a strange dog, try to capture or keep track of the dog or report it to law-enforcement officials. If the attacker lives for 10 days after biting your pet, you can eliminate rabies as a possible concern.

FIRST AID FOR BITE WOUNDS

1. Cleanse the wound thoroughly, immediately, and repeatedly with lots of soap and water.

2. Apply wound dressings (see pages 166–176 and 254–255).

3. Promptly get the patient to a veterinarian for treatment if the wound is serious.

If the bite was made by a possibly rabid animal

1. Cleanse and dress the wound as you would for an ordinary bite.

2. Take your pet to a veterinarian at once for treatment of the wound and for the appropriate rabies booster vaccination. Treatment is invariably effective in previously vaccinated patients; it is

highly effective in unvaccinated patients that are treated promptly and properly.

3. Notify your physician and public-health authorities—especially if humans are bitten, too!

Closed Wounds

CAUSES

Forceful impact with external objects—as in automobile accidents, falls, or severe blows—and untreated fractures.

SIGNS AND SYMPTOMS

1. Bleeding from natural body openings. Although there is no break in the skin or mucous membranes and blood is not lost through the skin, blood may pass from the mouth, rectum, etc. Since these wounds are closed, infection is uncommon. Usually there is internal bleeding and tissue damage. Injury can occur to any part of the body. It may be minor or extensive, with much physical damage to major organs or tissue systems.

2. Local pain.

3. Swelling.

4. Discoloration from internal bruising.

5. Deformity of a limb from fracture or (possibly) dislocation.

6. Pain and restlessness that seem exaggerated in terms of apparent injury.

7. Blood in the urine, feces, saliva, or in vomited food.

8. Bleeding from the ears or eyes.

9. Wobbly stance or inability to stand.

10. Coma, depression, or unconsciousness.

11. Signs of shock: collapse, cold face and extremities, pale tongue and mouth, rapid pulse (more than 120 per minute—see pages 189–191 and Figure 2, page 16), weak pulse, and rapid breathing (see pages 37–42 for details on shock).

FIRST AID FOR CLOSED WOUNDS

PRINCIPLES AND PROCEDURES

1. Maintain an open airway.

2. Examine the animal for fractures, bruises, or other obvious signs of injury.

3. Treat the animal for shock (see pages 39–41).

4. Immobilize any areas that could involve a fracture, severe sprain, or dislocation (see pages 108–113).

5. Do not give anything by mouth.

6. Transport the patient promptly to a veterinary hospital. Move the patient carefully, in a flat, secure position (see pages 148–149).

7. Treat with cold compresses if the closed wound is a small bruise. Apply compresses for 10 to 15 minutes every few hours. Do this soon after the injury, to reduce internal bleeding and prevent swelling of the tissue.

PREVENTION OF WOUNDS

Any accident may cause bruises, wounds, or fractures in pets. Animals are like children in that they are impetuous, do not think about consequences, and are often out of control. Accident prevention therefore involves attention to proper training and adequate control. This means voice, as well as leash, control.

1. Do not allow your pet to run free unless it is within your sight and under absolute control. When traveling in a busy area, keep the animal on a leash or carry it in your arms or in a carrier. A dog can easily be trained to stay within the confines of a yard if you are persistent. Dogs and cats are territorial animals and are

happy within the bounds of their home territory—whether it is a room, a pen, a yard, or a whole neighborhood. However, the possibility of an accident increases with the size of the territory.

2. A pet traveling in an automobile should never be allowed to ride with its head outside the window since foreign material may get in its eyes or strike its head. A pet should also be prevented from sitting on seats or leaning over the door, as sudden stops or swerves could pitch the animal out of the car. Sudden motions may cause injuries to a pet inside the car unless it is riding on the floor or in a "cat box." Train your pet to ride on the floor away from the driver's area.

3. Never allow your dog to chase cars. This is a prime cause of animal injuries. Every time a car "gets away," the dog is proud of its accomplishment—having chased off the invading machine— and this reinforces the bad habit. You can sometimes break a dog of the habit by having a stranger to the pet slow his car and throw ten or twelve small, empty tin cans at the chasing dog. The noise, clatter, and startling effect of this barrage will "defeat" the dog and perhaps teach it a lesson. Repeat if necessary.

An alternate method is to tie 40 to 50 feet of light nylon cord to your dog's collar; allow the dog to run after a car, and in the midst of the chase, pull back hard on the cord, jerking the dog sharply off its feet.

Still another simple method is to tie a short length of pipe to the dog's collar. The pipe should hang down just far enough to interfere with the dog's running. The frustration should discourage chasing.

If you cannot keep your pet confined, one of the above methods should work. Failure to resolve the problem inevitably results in an accident.

4. Do not allow your dog or cat access to high areas from which it may fall—window sills, fire escapes, or steep cliffs.

5. Keep pets out of store rooms, tool sheds, garages, and garbage areas where sharp instruments or chemicals are stored. A pet may walk in spilled chemicals (e.g., antifreeze, leaking from a

car), lick its feet, and thus be poisoned. It may also fall against a sharp implement or step on glass, a nail, or a jagged piece of metal and cut itself.

6. Prevent contact with stray animals. Most pets will defend their home territory against strangers, and severe fights can develop. Also, parasites and infectious diseases can be transmitted between animals even during friendly encounters.

6.

Shock

Definition

Shock is an acute failure of the peripheral circulation (the blood supply to the tissues of vital organs). It is a life-threatening condition that may result from the depression of any one of many vital functions.

Causes

Severe injury is the most common cause of shock in animals, but massive bleeding, acute body-fluid loss (as in vomiting, diarrhea, or wound drainage from burns), poisoning, infection, heart failure, and obstruction to breathing may also produce shock.

Shock develops when there is a malfunction of the circulatory system. Blood supply to the tissues is provided by three elements working together. This system can be compared to that of water supply.

1. The heart—a pump.
2. Blood vessels—pipes.
3. Blood—water.

Just as the supply of water to the house faucet depends on proper functioning of all three components, so the circulation of blood to the cells and organs of the body requires healthy cooperation of the heart, blood vessels, and blood. The circulatory system provides oxygen and nutrients and takes away waste products. If the heart does not function well, no blood circulates. If the vessels are clogged or broken, the blood supply cannot get through. And of course, if there is too little blood in the system it cannot supply the needy areas—even if the heart and vessels are normal.

In the treatment or prevention of shock, we direct all our efforts toward maintaining effective circulation. The body automatically attempts to do this

1. By speeding up the heartbeat.

2. By constricting the small blood vessels so blood is forced into major vessels, which supply the vital organs deep inside the body.

3. By increasing respiration in an attempt to increase the oxygen supply to the body parts deprived of oxygen as a result of the poor circulation.

These factors explain some of the signs and symptoms one sees in a shock patient.

Signs and Symptoms

1. Weakness, collapse, coma, and unconsciousness. These are caused by a poor blood supply to the brain; as the animal becomes less responsive the seriousness of the condition increases.

2. Pale color of the mouth, lips, and eyelids. This is caused by vascular (blood-vessel) constriction in these areas as the body attempts to send the decreased amount of blood to more vital areas.

3. Coolness of the skin and legs to the touch. For the reasons given above, there is poor blood supply to the skin, which makes it cool. The body temperature, as taken by rectal thermometer (see pages 187–189), may be low.

4. Rapid heart rate (pulse). It may be over 140 per minute, and may be difficult to feel (see pages 189–191 and Figure 2, page 16) and hard to count. The increased rate is an attempt to improve the pumping efficiency of the heart; the faintness is an indication of weak heart action.

5. Rapid respiratory rate (over 40 per minute) and breathing

may be shallow and irregular. The increased rate is an attempt to provide more oxygen to the deprived body tissues.

6. Sunken, fixed, and staring eyes. The pupils may be dilated. These are grave signs, which indicate that serious or fatal consequences are probable.

FIRST AID FOR SHOCK

PRINCIPLES

1. Eliminate or compensate for the cause of shock.

2. Maintain effective circulation.

3. Maintain adequate ventilation (oxygen to the body).

4. Maintain the body temperature.

5. Do not aggravate injuries.

6. Move the patient promptly, gently, and safely to a veterinary hospital.

PROCEDURES

1. Eliminate the cause of shock.

   a. Maintain an open airway—be sure it is free of obstruction. Give artificial respiration if necessary (see pages 14–16).

   b. Stop or control bleeding (as described on pages 23–28).

   c. Give cardiac massage if necessary (see page 4).

   d. Remove the patient from the source of electric shock, poison, or asphyxia.

   e. Restore body heat.

2. Maintain effective circulation. Keep the head as low as the rest of the body if the patient is unconscious. Lowering the head uses gravity to aid blood returning to the heart and thus improves circulation. Gently massage the legs and muscles. If the patient is restless, keep it in a horizontal position, wrapped in blankets for the dual purpose of restraint and conserving body heat.

3. Maintain adequate ventilation. Get the patient into fresh air, clear the mouth and throat of any fluids or obstructions, pull the tongue forward out of the mouth so that it does not interfere with breathing. Observe the patient's breathing; if it is slow and irregular or has stopped, start artificial respiration immediately (see pages 14–16 and Figure 1, page 15).

4. Maintain body temperature. Conserve body heat, but do not use external heating devices. An animal in shock has poor skin circulation and can easily be burned by a heat lamp or heating pad. Keep the patient in a warm room (or a well-heated car while it is being transported to the hospital) and help retain body heat by wrapping the animal firmly in warm blankets.

5. Do not aggravate injuries. Bandage, pad, or splint any fracture or extensive wound (see pages 109–111 and 166–176) as necessary and protect the injured part from movement, exposure, and contamination. Avoid factors that add to the pain or fright of the patient.

6. Transport the patient promptly to a veterinary hospital. It is imperative that you perform the simple emergency procedures listed above, but do not try to clean the patient or use more detailed treatment methods. With severe shock, *time* is vitally important. *Early* administration of large amounts of intravenous fluids is the most valuable single treatment—and this must be done at the hospital. This treatment becomes progressively less effective as time passes; so delay of a few minutes may greatly diminish the patient's chances of recovery.

Don't delay! Get to the hospital promptly, but drive safely.

7. Use the following procedures if veterinary help is too distant, unavailable, or unobtainable for several hours.

    a. Administer fluids orally, as for burns, if the patient is conscious. Give the patient 1 to 4 ounces (depending on the size of the patient) of a tepid water solution, containing ½ teaspoon salt and ½ teaspoon of bicarbonate of soda per quart of water. Readminister this solution every 30 minutes for a total of 4 or 5 doses. *Do not* give this solution, or anything else by mouth if the animal is unconscious, having convulsions, or vomiting. The patient may inhale the liquid into the lungs or aggravate a stomach injury.

    b. Clean and properly dress any wound (see pages 23–29).

    c. Take the pulse and breathing rate (pages 189–191) every 30 minutes and record them. Observe the patient for new symptoms or changes in consciousness. Look for the presence of blood in the patient's urine, stool, or saliva. Observations of this kind will be helpful to the veterinarian who eventually treats your pet.

    d. Keep the patient still. Do not let your pet struggle or walk around even if it appears to be recovering. Quiet, rest, and warmth are essential.

Prevention

1. The best way to prevent shock is by preventing serious accidents. This involves good pet control.

2. The practical time to prevent shock is when your pet has been injured but is not yet *in* shock. At such a time, the following steps are helpful.

    a. Stop bleeding promptly.

    b. Do not aggravate injuries by movement or actions that

will cause pain or fright (especially in the case of fractures).

c. Keep the patient lying down and quiet.
d. Avoid exposure to cold and dampness.
e. Conserve body heat with blankets.

7.

Poisoning

Each year, thousands of animals are accidentally—or even purposely—poisoned. Pets are like children. They are curious, and they commonly mouth or chew strange objects. If they find the taste appealing, they swallow all sorts of foreign and toxic materials. These may be medicines, cleaning agents, plant and insect sprays, ornamental plants, exotic foods, garbage, or dead animals. In addition, many animals clean themselves by licking and in this way swallow any toxic material that adheres to their coat and paws. Pet owners must assume responsibility for safeguarding their pets from exposure to needless danger.

Definition

A poison is a substance that produces bodily harm or causes death when it is introduced into the body or onto the skin surface.

Poisoning occurs in four ways:
1. By ingestion (through the mouth).
2. By inhalation (breathed in through the mouth or nose).
3. By absorption (through the skin).
4. By injection (directly into the bloodstream or tissues).

Signs and Symptoms

Signs of poisoning vary widely. Since pets can communicate their distress only through their actions, our observations must translate their symptoms.

We can suspect poisoning if we observe:

1. Pets chewing or contacting material of a questionable nature.

2. Spilled, opened, or chewed containers of medicine, chemicals, garbage, spoiled food, etc.

3. Material on an animal's coat, mouth, or feet that could be toxic.

4. An abnormal odor about the pet's breath or body.

5. Burns or painful areas on the skin or mouth parts.

6. A sudden change in bodily functions, such as vomiting, diarrhea, difficult breathing, or abdominal pain.

Symptoms vary widely, depending on the nature of the poison and the way it has entered the body.

1. Poisons entering by mouth often cause stomach and bowel symptoms, such as cramps and abdominal pain, followed by vomiting and diarrhea. The animal may drool, act weak, and breathe slowly.

2. Poisons that are inhaled often cause coughing and sneezing, shortness of breath, and blueness of the lining of the mouth. Severe labored breathing may also develop, and in serious cases, breathing may stop.

3. Poisons that are absorbed following skin contact cause redness, pain, and peeling of the affected area. Severe irritation of the eyes and mouth may also occur.

4. Poisons that are injected under the skin (insect bites or snakebites) produce pain and swelling at the point of injection. Many injected poisons quickly produce general effects on breathing, circulation, and on the pet's nervous system.

Sources and Examples

1. Animals often swallow poisons when they are allowed access to spilled medicines and chemicals (antifreeze, oil, tar, cleaning fluids, polishes, insecticides, weed killers, fertilizers, paints, solvents; medicines, drugs, or chemicals transferred from original con-

tainers; alkalies, acids, etc.) Pets may also walk in these substances and then lick them off their feet. For a list of potentially dangerous common household items see pages 49–53.

Mixing over-the-counter drugs with prescription items ordered by your veterinarian is another possible cause of poisoning. Drug interactions are very complex. *Always be certain your veterinarian knows all the facts about any and all medications that your pet has received recently.*

Many poisonous plants are readily available to pets. Some animals develop abnormal habits of chewing or ingesting plants and grass. Individual dogs may become "grazers" and eat quite large amounts of harmless lawn grass with apparent gusto. This is usually insignificant. However, if the grass has been sprayed with insecticidal, fungicidal, or herbicidal chemicals, the toxic potential may be great.

Few pet owners realize how many common ornamental house plants can produce toxic reactions in pets. Pets may chew the plants, often as a result of boredom. These habits should be stopped *immediately*. The toxic ingredients in poisonous plants vary widely in their effect on the pet, so specific treatment also varies. The general measures of treatment in "First Aid For Ingested Poisons" (pages 53–55) are effective in many cases, but specific treatment requires veterinary assistance. For a list of potentially dangerous ornamental plants see pages 46–49.

2. Pets inhale poisons when they are exposed to fumes from cleaning fluid, gasoline, kerosene, lacquer thinner, airplane glue, automobile or heater exhaust, smoke, or refrigerators with gas leaks (see table on pages 49–53).

3. Poisons that commonly come in contact with the pet's skin include paint solvents, kerosene, tar, insecticides, strong soaps, acids, and alkalies (see table on pages 49–53). These may all produce severe local skin reactions.

4. Injectable poisons usually enter the pet's body as a result of bites from poisonous snakes, spiders, and insects (see Figure 8, page 63).

Potentially Dangerous Plants—Toxic Effects and Early Symptoms

COMMON NAME	SCIENTIFIC NAME	EARLY SYMPTOMS

I. Oral, Pharyngeal, and Esophageal Irritants

COMMON NAME	SCIENTIFIC NAME	EARLY SYMPTOMS
Alocasia	*Alocasia spp.*	Salivation and edema
Caladium	*Caladium spp.*	(swelling)
Calla lily	*Zantedeschia acthiopica*	
Dumbcane	*Dieffenbachia spp.*	
Elephant's-ear	*Colocasia spp.*	
Green dragon, Oregon root	*Arisaema dracontium*	
Jack-in-the-pulpit, Indian turnip	*Arisaema triphyllum*	
Malanga	*Xanthosoma spp.*	
Philodendron	*Philodendron spp.*	
Skunk cabbage	*Symplocarpus foetidus*	

II. Gastric Irritants

Amaryllis	*Amaryllis spp.*	Immediate nausea and
Daffodil	*Narcissus spp.*	vomiting
Wisteria	*Wisteria spp.*	

III. Intestinal Irritants

Balsam pear	*Momordica charantia*	Salivation, immediate
English ivy	*Hedera helix*	nausea and vomiting,
Horse chestnut, buckeye	*Aesculus spp.*	abdominal pain, and diarrhea
Mock orange	*Poncirus spp.*	
Pongam	*Pongamia pinnata*	
Rain tree, monkey pod	*Samonia samen*	
Soapberry	*Sapindus saponaria*	
Yam bean	*Pachyrhizus erosus*	
Bloodberry, baby-pepper	*Rivina humilis*	Immediate nausea and vomiting, abdominal
Daphne, spurge laurel	*Daphne spp.*	pain, and diarrhea
Iris, flag	*Iris spp.*	
Lords-and-ladies	*Arum spp.*	
Pokeweed	*Phytolacca americana*	
American yew	*Taxus canadensis*	Immediate nausea and
English yew	*Taxus baccata*	vomiting, abdominal
Japanese yew	*Taxus cuspidata*	pain, pupil dilation, and
Western yew	*Taxus breviflora*	irregular heartbeat
Baneberry	*Actaea spp.*	Immediate vomiting,
Clematis	*Clematis spp.*	diarrhea, and rash.

IV. Miscellaneous Gastrointestinal Irritants and Cathartics

Bird-of-paradise bush	*Poinciana gilliesi*	Immediate nausea and vomiting, abdominal
Buckthorn	*Rhamnus spp.*	pain, and diarrhea;

COMMON NAME	SCIENTIFIC NAME	EARLY SYMPTOMS
Candlenut	*Aleurites spp.*	nervous or kidney
Christmas candle	*Pedilanthus tithymaloides*	involvement follows
Clusia	*Clusia rosea*	with some plants in
Common box	*Buxus sempervirens*	this group
English holly	*Ilex aquifolium*	
Euonymus	*Euonymus spp.*	
Honeysuckle	*Lonicera tatarica*	
Poinsettia	*Euphorbia pulcherrima*	
Privet	*Ligustrum spp.*	
Yellow allamanda	*Allamanda cathartica*	

V. Delayed Gastrointestinal Effects

Black locust	*Robinia pseudoacacia*	Delayed vomiting,
Castor bean	*Ricinus communis*	abdominal pain,
Coral plant	*Jatropha multifida*	diarrhea (followed by
Rosary pea,		constipation with
precatory bean	*Abrus precatorius*	Robinia), depression or
Sandbox tree,		coma, and low blood
monkey pistol	*Hura crepitans*	pressure
Bittersweet woody		
nightshade	*Solanum dulcamara*	Delayed vomiting,
Chalice vine	*Solandra spp.*	abdominal pain,
Ground cherry	*Physalis spp.*	diarrhea, and dry oral
Jerusalem cherry	*Solanum pseudo-capsicum*	mucous membranes in Cestrum; cardiac
Jessamine	*Cestrum spp.*	activity with Jerusalem
Potato	*Solanum tuberosum*	cherry
Garden sorrel	*Rumex acetosa*	Delayed vomiting,
Rhubarb	*Rheum rhaponticum*	abdominal pain,
Virginia creeper	*Psedera quinquefolia*	diarrhea, depression or coma
Autumn erocus	*Colchicum spp.*	Delayed vomiting,
Glory lily	*Gloriosa spp.*	abdominal pain, and diarrhea

VI. Cardiovascular Disturbances

Foxglove	*Digitalis purpurea*	Immediate nausea and
Lily of the valley	*Convallaria majalis*	vomiting, abdominal
Oleander	*Nerium spp.*	pain, slow and
Yellow oleander	*Thevetia peruviana*	irregular heartbeat
Aconite, monks-hood		Immediate nausea,
Larkspur	*Aconitum napeilus*	tremors and convul-
	Delphinium spp.	sion, slow and ir-
Western monks-hood		regular heartbeat, and
	Aconitum columbianum	difficult breathing

VII. Nicotinelike Action

Cardinal flower,		Salivation, immediate
Indian tobacco	*Lobelia spp.*	nausea and vomiting,
Golden chain	*Laburnum anagyroides*	and rapid heartbeat

COMMON NAME	SCIENTIFIC NAME	EARLY SYMPTOMS
Kentucky coffee tree	*Gymnocladus dioica*	
Mescal bean	*Sophora spp.*	
Poison hemlock	*Conium maculatum*	
Tobacco	*Nicotiana spp.*	

VIII. Atropine Action

Angel's-trumpet	*Datura arborea*	Dilated pupils, dry
Belladonna, deadly		mouth, difficult breath-
nightshade	*Atropa belladonna*	ing, fever, and rapid
Henbane	*Hyoscyamus niger*	heartbeat
Jessamine	*Cestrum spp.*	
Jimson weed,		
thorn apple	*Datura spp.*	
Matrimony vine	*Lycium halimifolium*	

IX. Convulsants

Chinaberry	*Melia azedarach*	Convulsions
Coriaria	*Coriaria supp.*	
Moonseed	*Menispermum canadense*	
Nux vomica	*Strychnos nux-vomica*	
Water hemlock	*Cicuta maculata*	

X. Behavioral Alterants, Hallucinogens

Marijuana	*Cannabis sativa*	Abnormal emotional or
Morning-glory	*Ipomoea spp.*	dispositional effects
Nutmeg	*Myristica fragrans*	
Periwinkle	*Vinca rosea*	
Peyote, mescal	*Lophophora williamsii*	

XI. Cyanogenetic Action

Apricot, almond,		Vomiting, stupor, difficult
peach, cherry,		breathing, and coma;
chokecherry,		bright red venous
wild cherry	*Prunus spp.*	blood
Hydrangea	*Hydrangea macrophylla*	
Japanese plum	*Eriobotrya japonica*	

XII. Contact Irritants or Mechanical Injury

Nettle	*Urtica chamaedryoides*	Salivation, vomiting, slow
Nettle	*Laportea canadensis*	and irregular heart-
Nettle spurge	*Cnidoscolus stimulosus*	beat, difficult breathing
Stinging nettle,		
bull nettle	*Urtica dioica*	
Blackberry	*Rubus spp.*	Inflamed mouth, con-
Burdock	*Arctium lappa*	junctivitis, abscesses,
Cacti	*Numerous genera*	fistulous tracts, re-
Carolina night-		duced performance,
shade	*Solanum carolinense*	hemorrhage, or
		lameness

COMMON NAME	SCIENTIFIC NAME	EARLY SYMPTOMS
Foxtail	*Setaria spp.*	
Goathead	*Tribulus terrestris*	
Honey locust	*Gleditsia triacanthos*	
Needlegrass	*Stipa spp.*	
Sandbur	*Cenchrus pauciflorus*	
Tripleawn	*Aristida spp.*	
Wild barley	*Hordeum spp.*	
Wild brome	*Bromus spp.*	

Adapted from K. F. Lampe and R. Fagerstrom, *Plant Toxicity and Dermatitis: A Manual for Physicians* (Baltimore: The Williams and Wilkins Co., 1968).

Some Chemical Products Hazardous to Pets

ARTS AND CRAFTS SUPPLIES

Antiquing Agents
Methyl ethyl ketone
Turpentine

Oil Paints and Tempera Paints
Pigment salts of lead, arsenic, copper,
and cadmium

Pencils, Indelible
Crystal violet

PHOTOGRAPHIC SUPPLIES

Developers
Borates
Bromides
Iodides
Thiocyanates

Fixatives
Sodium thiosulfate

Hardeners
Aluminum chloride
Formaldehyde

AUTOMOTIVE AND MACHINERY PRODUCTS

Antifreeze, Fuel System De-icer
Ethylene glycol
Isopropyl alcohol
Methanol
Rust inhibitors
 a. Borates
 b. Chromates
 c. Zinc chloride

Brake Fluids
Butyl ethers of ethylene glycol and
related glycols

Ethyl ethers of ethylene glycol and
related glycols
Methyl ethers of ethylene glycol and
related glycols

Carburetor Cleaners
Cresol
Ethylene dichloride

Corrosion Inhibitors
Borates
Sodium chromate
Sodium nitrate

Some Chemical Products Hazardous to Pets

Engine and Motor Cleaners
Cresol
Ethylene dichloride
Methylene chloride

Frost Removers
Ethylene glycol
Isopropyl alcohol

Lubricants
Barium compounds
Isopropyl alcohol
Kerosene
Lead compounds
Stoddard solvent

Motor Fuel
Gasoline

Kerosene
Tetraethyl lead

Radiator Cleaners
Boric acid
Oxalic acid
Sodium chromate

Shock Absorber Fluids
Petroleum ether

Tire Repair
Benzene

Windshield Washer
Ethylene glycol
Isopropyl alcohol
Methyl alcohol

CLEANERS, DISINFECTANTS, SANITIZERS

Cleaners, Bleaches, Polishes
Ammonium hydroxide
Benzene
Carbon tetrachloride
Hydrochloric acid
Methyl alcohol
Naphtha
Nitrobenzene
Oxalic acid
Phosphoric acid
Sodium fluoride
Sodium or potassium hydroxide
Sodium hypochlorite
Sodium perborate

Sulfuric acid
Trichloroethane
Turpentine

Disinfectants, Sanitizers
Acids
Alkalies
Hypochlorites
Iodophors
Paradichlorobenzene
Phenol, Cresols
Phenyl mercuric acetate
Pine oil
Quaternary ammonium

HEALTH AND BEAUTY AIDS

Athlete's Foot
Caprylic acid
Copper
Propionic acid
Sodium
Undecylenic acid
Zinc salts

Bath Preparations
Bath oils
Perfume
Sodium lauryl sulfate
Trisodium phosphate

Corn Removers
Phenoxyacetic acid
Salicylic acid

Deodorants and Antiperspirants
Alcohol
Aluminum chloride

Diet Pills
Amphetamines
Diuretics
Thyroid hormone

Eye Makeup
Boric acid
Peach kernel oil, q.s.

Hair Preparations
Cadmium chloride
Cupric chloride
Dyes, tints

Some Chemical Products Hazardous to Pets

Ferric chloride
Lead acetate
Permanent wave lotions
Pyrogallol
Silver nitrate
Thioglycolic acid

Headache
Aspirin
Phenacetin

Laxatives
Irritant or Stimulant Laxatives
  Aloes
  Aloin
  Cascara sagrada

Liniments
Camphor
Chloroform
Oil of wintergreen (methyl salicylate)
Pine oil
Turpentine

Nailetics
Acetone
Alcohol
Benzene
Ethyl acetate
Nail enamel
Nail polish
Nail polish remover
Toluene
Tricresyl phosphate

Ointments
Benzoic acid
Borates
Caprylic acid
Menthol
Mercury compounds
Oil of wintergreen (methyl salicylate)
Phenols
Salicylic acid

Perfumes, Toilet Waters, and Colognes
Alcohol
Essential oils
Floral oils
Perfume essence

Shampoos
Sodium lauryl sulfate
Triethanolamine dodecyl sulfate

Shaving Lotions
Alcohol
Boric acid

Somnolents (Sleeping Pills)
Barbiturates
Bromides

Stimulants
Amphetamine
Caffeine

Suntan Lotions
Alcohol
Tannic acid and derivatives

PAINTS AND RELATED PRODUCTS

Caulking Compounds
Barium
Chlorinated biphenyl
Chromium
Lead
Mineral spirits
Petroleum distillate
Xylene

Driers
Cobalt compounds
Iron compounds
Manganese compounds
Vanadium compounds
Zinc compounds

Lacquer Thinners
Aliphatic hydrocarbons
Butyl acetate
Butyl alcohol
Toluene

Paint
Arsenic oxide
Coal tar
Cuprous oxide
Lead chromate
Petroleum ether
Pine oil
Red lead oxide
Zinc chromate

Some Chemical Products Hazardous to Pets

Paint Brush Cleaners
Benzene
Kerosene
Naphthas

Paint and Varnish Cleaners
Ethylene dichloride
Kerosene
Naphthalene
Trisodium phosphate

Paint and Varnish Removers
Flammable
  Benzene
  Cresols
  Phenols
  Toluene

Nonflammable
  Methylene chloride
  Toluene
Preservatives
Brush
  Kerosene
  Turpentine
Canvas
  2-Chlorophenylphenol
  Pentachlorophenol
Floor
  Magnesium fluorosilicate
Wood
  Copper naphthenate
  Copper oleate
  Mineral spirits
  Pentachlorophenol
  Zinc naphthenate

PEST CONTROL

Birds
Endrin
Toluidine

Fungicides
Captan
Copper compounds
Maneb
Mercurials
Pentachlorophenol
Thiram
Zineb

Insects and Spiders
Baygon
Carbaryl
Chlordane
Diazinon
Dichlorvos
Kelthane
Mirex
Paradichlorobenzene
Pyrethrins

Rotenone
Toxaphene

Lawn and Garden Weeds
Arsenic
Chlordane
Dacthal
Pentachlorophenol
Trifluralin
2,4-D

Rats, Mice, Gophers, Moles
Arsenic
Barium carbonate
Dicoumarol
Phosphorus
Sodium fluoroacetate
Strychnine
Thallium (rare)
Warfarin
Zinc phosphide

Snails, Slugs
Metaldehyde

SAFETY PRODUCTS

Fire Extinguishers
Liquid Fire Extinguishers
  Carbon tetrachloride
Miscellaneous Fire Extinguishers
  Methylbromide

Powder Extinguishers
  Borax compounds

Nonskid Products
Stoddard solvent
Methyl ethyl ketone

Some Chemical Products Hazardous to Pets

SOLVENTS

Alcohols

Chlorinated Solvents
Carbon tetrachloride
Methylene chloride
Orthodichlorobenzene
Trichloroethylene

Esters
Amyl acetate
Ethyl acetate
Isopropyl acetate
Methyl acetate

Hydrocarbons
Aromatics, chiefly benzene, toluene,
   and xylene
Naphthenes

Ketones
Acetone
Methyl ethyl ketone

Other Common Solvents
Aniline
Carbon disulphide
Cresylic acid
Kerosene
Mineral spirits
Phenols
Turpentine

From Gary D. Osweiler, D.V.M., "Some Chemical Products Hazardous to Pets."

FIRST AID FOR INGESTED (SWALLOWED) POISONS

Like food, ingested poisons remain in the stomach a short while before they pass into the intestines for absorption. Once absorbed, the problems of treatment are far more difficult.

PRINCIPLES

1. Remove ingested poisons before they can be absorbed (induce vomiting).

2. Prevent absorption of poisons that cannot be removed.

3. Neutralize or detoxify poisons that remain in the stomach or intestines.

4. Give specific antidotes, which will counteract the effects of the poison in the animal's body.

5. Give general supportive treatment to combat the effects of the absorbed poison.

PROCEDURES

1. Remove the source of poisoning so the animal cannot ingest any more.

2. Dilute an ingested acid, alkali, or petroleum product (such as gasoline or kerosene) with milk or vegetable oil—but *do not* induce vomiting. *Get the patient to a veterinary hospital at once.*

3. Induce vomiting if a corrosive substance such as mentioned above was *not* involved. Do this by giving 1 or 2 teaspoons of hydrogen peroxide by mouth every 5 to 10 minutes for a total of 3 or 4 doses or until vomiting occurs (see pages 192–193 and 252).

4. Save the vomitus for evaluation later, and save the label and/or container of the chemical or drug. Present both of these to the veterinarian for identification; they will help guide him as to specific treatment.

5. Get to a veterinarian quickly. If this is not possible and you know the specific antidotes (from the label), give these after the animal has vomited.

6. If you do not know the specific antidotes, dilute the poison (after vomiting has stopped) by giving water or milk—preferably mixed with several teaspoonsful of *activated* or medical charcoal (available at most drugstores). Consider the use of general antidotes.

7. If the patient is unconscious, do not attempt to give anything by mouth. Get the patient to the hospital promptly.

8. Observe breathing and give artificial respiration if necessary (see pages 14–16).

9. Keep the patient warm (wrap in a blanket) and keep its head lowered so that fluids in the mouth drain out and are not inhaled.

GENERAL ANTIDOTES

Containers of household chemicals usually have labels that include a specific antidote for that substance. If you do not have this information, you may be able to use one of the following common items:

For	*Use*
General poisons, to prevent absorption	Several teaspoons of activated charcoal or kaolin mixture, with large amounts of water or milk (page 252).
Acids	Antacids, such as milk of magnesia or baking soda (page 253).
Alkalies	Vinegar, lemon juice. Dilute with equal parts of water and flood skin or give 1 to 5 teaspoons orally.
Severe depression	Strong tea or coffee. Give 1 to 5 teaspoons orally.
Laxative effect to hasten material through the intestines	Milk of magnesia (page 253).
Diluting the poison and stimulating its removal by increasing urination	Copious amounts of lukewarm water, milk, or weak tea.
Coating the intestines to slow absorption	Milk, vegetable oil, kaolin, milk of bismuth, egg whites. These can be given freely, but a dose of 1 to 3 tablespoons is reasonable for many animals.

10. If the animal is very excitable or is convulsing, do not try to give anything by mouth and do not try to induce vomiting. Wrap the animal in a blanket and get to the hospital promptly.

11. Have someone telephone the veterinary hospital to give them advance notice of your plight and flight. Details given to the hospital should include: your name, the pet's species and age, the type of poison it ingested, symptoms you have observed, first aid steps you have taken, and the time you expect to arrive at the hospital.

FIRST AID FOR INHALED POISONS

Gases that can be injurious to animals include smoke; heated gases (from fire); carbon monoxide; toxic fumes from burning insulation, plastic materials, and upholstery; heating or cooking gas; and freon, ammonia, and other refrigerants.

PRINCIPLES AND PROCEDURES

1. Get the animal out of the contaminated area into clean air.

2. Provide artificial respiration if necessary (see pages 14–16 and Figure 1, page 15).

3. Clear airway. Loosen tight collar, remove any foreign material from mouth or throat (see pages 70–71).

4. Get the patient to a source of oxygen (hospital) promptly. Animals with carbon monoxide poisoning usually have cherry-red lips and tongue and are weak and dizzy. They will die if oxygen is not obtained immediately.

5. Be most cautious about rescuing pets at the risk of your own life. If you must rescue an animal from a contaminated area, hold your breath, dash into the building or room, open doors and windows, and go right out again without breathing. Then make a second trip for the pet. Do not linger! It is better to leave such

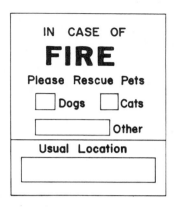

FIGURE 7. *A fire notice.* Posting a notice such as this may enable an emergency squad to rescue your pet(s). Similar decals may be obtained from Friends of Animals, Inc., Dept. 516, 11 West 60 Street, New York, N.Y. 10023.

rescue attempts to an emergency squad, especially if fire is involved. *Never go into a burning building!*

6. Post a notice on your door to advise rescue squads of the location of pets on the premises (see Figure 7).

FIRST AID FOR CONTACT POISONS

Pets very often are poisoned when they walk or roll in toxic materials. This will usually cause chemical burns to the portions of skin that have come into contact with the substance. The animal may also lick the substance off its coat and feet. After the poison is eaten, it will be absorbed into the animal's system and cause general symptoms. Pets may also be poisoned when hot or caustic liquids are spilled on them in kitchens or workshops.

An animal's coat is a mixed blessing; it protects against contact with poisonous plants (such as poison ivy and poison oak) but it will also hold some toxins, such as tar, paint, grease, and kerosene in contact with the skin for a prolonged period of time, thus accentuating the damage. (Pet owners should be aware that even though poison ivy and poison oak on an animal's coat do not bother the pet, they may cause a reaction in a human who contacts the pet and is sensitive to these plants.)

PRINCIPLES

1. Dilute and wash off the poison.

2. Use soap and water if indicated.

3. Do not use chemical solvents, such as gasoline, kerosene, paint remover, or any medication unless it has been specifically advised.

PROCEDURES

1. Use a hose, bathtub, or other device to provide huge quantities of plain water to dilute and remove the poisonous substance. Rinse the area affected for at least ten minutes.

2. Use a shampoo or soap and water to remove mildly greasy or water-insoluble solutions (such as latex paint).

3. Soak the animal's coat with milk to neutralize the effect of kerosene, gasoline, etc. You can also use vegetable oil in the same way. After thirty minutes wash the animal with soap and water to remove the oil or milk—and the poison. Mineral oil is another possible neutralizer, but it is much less soluble in soap and water and thus harder to wash off.

4. Road tar, which is soft in summer, commonly accumulates in large clumps between the toes or on the feet and legs of an animal. Use scissors to clip large masses off the affected hair coat. Soak smaller amounts thoroughly in vegetable oil, cover the area with a bandage, and leave it on overnight to allow the oil to penetrate the tar. By the next day, you can usually wash the tar out successfully

with a detergent and warm water. If necessary, repeat this procedure several times, until you have completely removed the tar.

5. The best way to remove oil-based paint is to allow it to dry and then clip off the paint-coated hair. Never use a paint remover. Also avoid turpentine and gasoline, as they are highly irritating. You can rub vegetable oil into the affected area and then wash gently with detergents.

6. Skunk-sprayed animals present a very special problem. The pungent secretion of the skunk's scent glands is a sticky, oily-waxy material that defies efforts at complete removal. It is especially irritating to the pet's eyes. Immediately flush the sprayed animal's eyes with huge amounts of plain warm water. Then apply drops of warm olive oil to the eyeball itself. This will help until you can obtain veterinary aid.

When the entire animal has been sprayed, soak the coat in plain tomato juice and allow it to remain on for several minutes. Then wash it off with soap and water.

You may also use dilute washes or rinses of a solution containing 1 tablespoon of household ammonia to 2 quarts of water as a final wash. Rinse this solution off promptly. Be careful to keep it out of the animal's eyes and ears and away from other sensitive parts. The patient may need daily baths of soap and water or occasional baths of ammonia and water for several days to further remove the scent. Even then, when the animal gets wet, there will be an odoriferous reminder of this recent experience.

FIRST AID FOR INJECTED POISONS

It is illegal for nonprofessional persons to possess syringes and needles without a prescription; so the possibility of poisoning by this sort of injection is remote. However, one should recognize that all animals (including people) occasionally react negatively to vaccines and other injected drugs. Most of these problems are allergic reactions. In these rare cases, veterinary aid is readily available (since the veterinarian has just administered the medication, specific antidotes and expert care are at hand).

Toxins are usually injected into the animal's body as the result of bites from insects, spiders, and poisonous snakes.

Insect Bites

Because pets cannot tell us the circumstances of their injuries, we must classify insect bites by the types of reactions they produce.

1. *Bites from bees, wasps, hornets, and yellowjackets* usually produce a large, flat, swollen area—a wheal—which occurs suddenly and is extremely painful. Bites are often on the animal's face or head. Repeated stings may cause the pet to develop an acute allergic (or anaphylactic) reaction, and difficult breathing and/or death are possible.

2. *Bites from fleas, mosquitos, lice, chiggers, and gnats* usually produce multiple, small, solid red pimples (papules), which itch intensely. The pet often licks and scratches itself severely, thus causing secondary injury to its own skin. Although generalized or severe reactions are rare, many dogs and cats develop a chronic allergic reaction to flea saliva. This causes generalized hair loss and thickened, reddened skin along the lower back, just in front of the tail.

Fleas may be the intermediate host, for some dog and cat tapeworms—as mosquitos are for the completion of the life cycle of heartworms. Control of these two pests is thus especially important to your pet's good health. (See pages 221–223.)

3. *Ticks* usually remain on the animal for relatively long periods of time, and they are often discovered as gray or brown, coffee-bean-sized objects fixed to the skin. They suck blood and are important transmitters of several blood diseases. They may cause "tick paralysis"; but the usual bite is a minor injury.

4. *Bites from spiders (including tarantulas) and scorpions* usually produce painful local reactions. These reactions to the venom and the lesions often progress to open sores that heal slowly.

Bites from the black widow spider and the brown recluse spider may produce generalized pain, nausea, chills and fever, painful cramps, and difficult breathing. Spiders are commonly found in wood and brush piles, seldom-used buildings, and basement areas. Tarantulas are rare in this country, but may be present in fruit-shipments from tropical areas.

FIRST AID FOR INSECT BITES

PRINCIPLES

   1. Remove the parasite.

   2. Cleanse the skin.

   3. Apply soothing, anti-inflammatory topical medication.

   4. Treat allergic reaction if necessary.

PROCEDURES: LOCAL REACTIONS

   1. Remove the insects by using flea or tick sprays or powders. Ticks must be removed in special ways. *Never hold a lighted cigarette to the ticks.* Soak them in tick spray, mineral oil, or alcohol, and after a few minutes gently tease them off the skin with fine tweezers. Try to remove the ticks with their heads intact. Place the ticks in a jar of alcohol to kill them and also to save them for identification by your veterinarian. Some of these insects live in houses, as well as outdoors, so proper identification is necessary to maintain control of the problem by exterminators or by your own measures. Get professional advice on this important aspect of insect control.

   2. Cleanse the affected areas gently with soap and water, wipe with alcohol, and dry. Remove the stinger if one is present. Cold

compresses—or wet compresses with Domeboro solution (available at most drugstores), sodium bicarbonate paste, or soothing lotions—should reduce the itching and swelling. More severe reactions should have veterinary care.

PROCEDURES: SYSTEMIC OR SEVERE REACTION

1. Apply ice packs if local swelling is severe. If a leg is involved, bandage it firmly between the swelling and the body to prevent spread of the poison.

2. Take the patient to a veterinary hospital immediately—delay can be serious.

3. Give artificial respiration if necessary (see pages 14–16 and Figure 1, page 15).

Snakebites

It is unusual for a snake to attack a pet. But if this does happen to your dog or cat, kill the snake (if you can do so safely) for later identification. Since most snakes are harmless and even beneficial, this suggestion applies particularly to those readers who live in areas with a high proportion of venomous reptiles (Australia, tropical and subtropical lands, and special locations within those areas).

The diagnosis of snakebite is usually based on the outward signs and symptoms, together with a history of probable exposure. For our purposes, snakes and their bites are divided into nonpoisonous and poisonous varieties.

Nonpoisonous snakes have no fangs; their bites leave tooth marks that look like scratches and/or multiple fine puncture wounds arranged in the shape of a U. The wounds are not especially painful and do not swell rapidly or extensively. Nonpoisonous snakes have eyes with round pupils, there is no pit or indentation between the eye and the nostril and they have a double row of plates beneath the tail (see Figure 8).

SNAKES

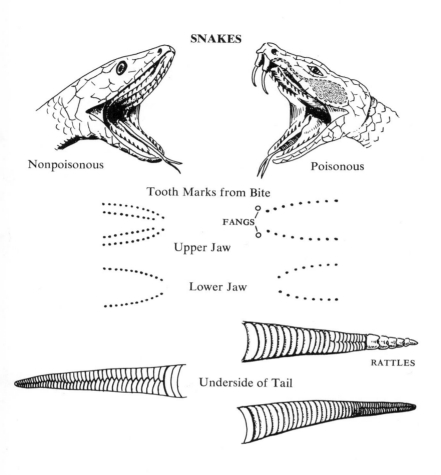

Nonpoisonous

Poisonous

Tooth Marks from Bite

FANGS

Upper Jaw

Lower Jaw

RATTLES

Underside of Tail

FIGURE 8. *Identifying features of poisonous and nonpoisonous snakes.* Note characteristics of the heads, undertails, and the tooth and fang marks in the bite wound.

Poisonous snakes in North America include the pit vipers (rattlesnakes, copperheads, and cottonmouth moccasins). These reptiles have large heads and two large fangs, which, in biting, produce distinct puncture wounds, with a few smaller tooth marks behind them. Because pet animals usually have heavy hair coats, the wounds may be difficult to find and identify. There is usually acute pain almost immediately after the bite, and there may be severe swelling, with bloody fluid oozing from the wounds.

Because of the dog's inquisitive and aggressive habits, snake-bites are usually found on the dog's face and forelegs. Cats may hunt and catch small nonpoisonous snakes, but they usually avoid large poisonous types. When a large snake bites a small animal, so much venom is injected into areas where absorption is rapid that toxic results are accentuated. The symptoms may rapidly progress from weakness and difficult breathing to shock and death.

Coral snakes are small and rare. They are occasionally found in the southeastern United States. They have small heads, round pupils, and double plates under their tails. However, these snakes are most easily recognized by their black noses and the red, yellow, and black rings around their bodies. Red and yellow rings always adjoin. Reactions to coral-snake bites are mild *locally,* but nervous signs, such as respiratory paralysis, convulsions, and coma develop rapidly. Many patients die from these bites.

FIRST AID FOR SNAKEBITES

PRINCIPLES

1. Reduce circulation in the area of the bite to delay the absorption of venom.

2. Remove venom from the bite wounds.

3. Cleanse and protect the wounds.

4. Support respiration and vital functions until veterinary aid can be provided.

PROCEDURES

1. Muzzle the animal, as it will resent your handling the painful wound.

2. If you are treating within 1 hour of the bite, and if the bite is on a leg, apply a tight 1-inch bandage around the leg between the swollen bite area and the body.

3. Use a sharp knife or razor blade and incise the fang wounds parallel to the long axis of the leg. Extend the wound ½ inch toward the toes.

4. If possible, suck wound with mouth to remove venom. Cleanse well with mild soap and water. Dry and apply ice packs to the wound. The ice should be contained in a cloth or plastic bag.

5. *Do not* give alcohol or a stimulant of any kind.

6. Get the patient to a veterinarian as soon as possible.

Toad Poisoning

Nine species of toads are reported to produce poisoning in dogs. These are found in gardens and fields in semitropical climates. Usually the dog playfully attacks the toad. The toad's salivary glands produce a potent toxin that produces severe symptoms when it contacts the mouth or eyes of the dog. The toxin may produce drooling, seizures, rapid heartbeat, and rapid breathing. Death may occur if prompt veterinary treatment is not obtained.

FIRST AID FOR TOAD POISONING

PRINCIPLES AND PROCEDURES

1. Wash the dog's face, eyes, and mouth with copious amounts of cool water (use a hose, if there is one available).

2. If the patient is unconscious, wrap it in a blanket to maintain body heat.

3. Transport to a veterinary hospital *at once*. Cases treated three to five or more hours after exposure may not respond well.

4. Give artificial respiration if necessary (see pages 14–16 and Figure 1, page 15).

Prevention

1. Keep medicines and chemicals in original containers and stored in a locked cabinet or closet.

2. Do not reuse containers that have held toxic agents.

3. Read labels and use drugs and chemicals only as directed. Observe the "outdated" warnings.

4. Properly dispose of old drugs and chemicals (flush them down the toilet).

5. Do not allow your animal pet to chew on plants, unknown objects, or garbage. This is for the animal's health—but preventing such behavior will also make your pet a more acceptable neighborhood citizen.

6. Keep your pet under control at all times. Wandering animals develop bad habits, and you may not know what difficulty your animal has caused or gotten into until it is too late to help.

7. Keep an animal first aid kit (page 145 and Figure 10, page 146) and a copy of this book available for quick reference.

Poison-Control Centers

Poison-control centers can be found in large metropolitan hospitals and in selected rural centers around the country. They maintain up-to-date data banks on poisons and current methods of treatment. When faced with a difficult poisoning problem, these centers, although designed to provide information about human poisoning, can be extremely helpful in providing information to help pets. Before you or your veterinarian call the poison-control center, be sure you know the name of the commercial product or agent involved in your pet's poisoning. (There are more than half a million commercial chemicals and household products on the market today.) Then the poison-control center can get the latest information on the toxic agent in the product and advise you of the best treatment method.

Call your local hospital or medical society to get the telephone number of the nearest poison-control center. Record this number in the front of this book *now*—before an emergency arises.

8.

Swallowed Foreign Objects
and Choking

Dogs and cats frequently mouth or chew objects for a number of reasons: out of curiosity, in an attempt to get rid of material in the mouth, to appreciate flavor, to clean their teeth, and out of sheer boredom. They may play with toys, balls, or sticks in a game with their owners. Like human babies, puppies and kittens have a developmental stage when they are teething (between the ages of 6 weeks and 6 months). Chewing on hard objects massages the gums and helps alleviate the discomfort of this normal process. Because of their natural inquisitiveness and their teething needs, young pets are more commonly involved with foreign-body problems. Perhaps our "senior citizen" pets have developed more common sense or just a more placid outlook on life.

Causes

1. A piece of stick or bone may become wedged between the teeth.

2. Sharp objects (needles, pins, or fishhooks; bone splinters from fish, chops, or chicken) may penetrate the tongue, throat, intestines, or rectum.

3. Round objects, that are small enough to go part way through the digestive tract, may become stuck in the throat, stomach, or small intestine. Stones, balls, nuts, pieces of bone, playthings, or even pieces of string or cloth may cause problems. Foreign bodies are most serious when they produce complete obstruction—espe-

cially in the back of the mouth, where they can interfere with breathing.

4. In rare cases foreign objects, such as sticks, may be introduced from the outside into an animal's ears, nose, rectum, or vagina by a cruel or sadistic person.

Signs and Symptoms

1. *In the mouth*
    a. Profuse drooling.
    b. Pawing at the mouth, rubbing the face on the ground.
    c. Continuous movements of the jaw and tongue.
    d. Choking, gagging, breathing in deep gasps (a foreign object caught at the back of the throat may cause asphyxia).
    e. Blueness of the tongue and mouth (caused by difficulty in breathing).
    f. Difficulty in swallowing (the animal usually wants to eat but will refuse any food offered—it just hurts to swallow).
2. *In the esophagus*
    a. Drooling and gulping.
    b. Refusal of food or immediate vomiting (if the animal attempts to eat).
3. *In the stomach or intestine*
    a. Abdominal pain and bloody vomitus (if the object is sharp).
    b. Profuse vomiting, depression, and shock (when a foreign object causes an intestinal obstruction—obtain prompt veterinary care, since surgical correction is usually needed).

    A foreign object may stay in the animal's stomach for a relatively long period and may cause little trouble except occasional vomiting. However, the digestive juices may react with an object such as a rubber ball and actually swell or distort it after a few days.

    Lead fishing sinkers left in the stomach for a long time may be partially absorbed and cause lead poisoning.

Other foreign bodies, such as bones or soft objects, may occasionally be digested and pass successfully out of the intestine with a bowel movement.

4. *In the rectum*
   a. Extreme pain when the animal strains for a bowel movement (caused by a sharp object).
   b. Blood in the stool, pet licking anus or area under the tail (from needles, safety pins, or hooks).

FIRST AID FOR FOREIGN-BODY OBSTRUCTIONS

PRINCIPLES

1. Attempt to remove the object if you can do so easily.

2. Do not give the animal anything by mouth.

3. Seek veterinary assistance at once if breathing is impaired.

Some foreign-body obstructions are less urgent emergencies and may be difficult to diagnose without sophisticated examination techniques. Do not delay seeking professional help if you suspect your pet has swallowed an unusual object. Long forceps, lights, and endoscopic equipment can often be inserted through the mouth to retrieve foreign objects from the esophagus and stomach.

PROCEDURES

FOREIGN BODIES IN THE TEETH OR MOUTH

1. Hold the animal securely. Wrap it in a heavy blanket—this is often safe, comfortable, and effective (see Figures 21 and 28, pages 158 and 164). Be sure the head is exposed for maximum visibility (see pages 154–159 and 163–165).

2. Open the mouth as wide as possible and inspect the teeth and throat.

3. Remove any visible foreign object with your fingers or with needle-nosed pliers or forceps—depending on which fits the area best. Bones, sticks, needles, and fishhooks may sometimes be easily removed. Do not pull on a thread or string—it may be attached to a needle and if so, can be used to trace the needle. However, this is a difficult procedure, and it requires veterinary equipment and skills. To extract a fishhook, you usually need to push it on through the tissue (lips or tongue), cut off the barbed hook with a wire cutter or pliers, and back the shank of the hook out. This may be painful and so may require anesthesia (if so, let your veterinarian handle it) or at least firm restraint. Porcupine quills may be removed from the mouth with forceps or pliers (see pages 247–248).

When the foreign material blocks the back of the throat or the larynx, it produces a life-threatening emergency. If possible, open the mouth, reach in with the fingers, and remove the obstruction. This is more easily accomplished—but more urgent—if the patient is unconscious.

4. The well-known Heimlich maneuver ("hug of life") for removing obstructions in human throats works for dogs and cats, too. The object is to compress the lower chest forcibly to raise air pressure inside the chest and "blow" the foreign material out of the throat or larynx. For the procedure:

   a. Place the patient on its side on a hard surface (the floor).

   b. Place both hands just behind the last rib and press down quickly and firmly. Release immediately and repeat rapidly several times. Try to direct the force of your hands slightly forward; this will make your efforts more effective.

   c. Have someone open the patient's mouth wide and attempt to retrieve material from the throat as you compress the chest.

   d. Once the airway is cleared, use artificial respiration (see pages 14–16 and Figure 1, page 15) until the animal breathes unassisted.

e. Seek veterinary aid promptly if your first efforts are not successful. Even if your first aid is effective, have your pet professionally examined for possible complications you may not see.

FOREIGN BODIES IN THE ESOPHAGUS, STOMACH, OR INTESTINES

1. Give nothing by mouth, since vomiting is usually present and eating and drinking aggravate the condition.

2. Seek professional help immediately. These are problems for your veterinarian.

3. Pad the object internally if you actually *see* your pet swallow a needle or pin and you cannot find it in the animal's mouth. This is a simple treatment, and it may be effective. Soak small pledgets of cotton (balls the size of a pencil eraser) in milk or meat broth and feed them to the patient. Your pet will usually eat the flavored cotton readily, and it will form a mass around the sharp object and guide it safely through the intestines. This procedure works especially well in cats. Of course, you should confine your pet for several days, examine each stool carefully until the object passes, and seek veterinary aid if stomach pain, lack of appetite, fever, or vomiting develop. X-ray examinations will locate these foreign bodies accurately if necessary.

FOREIGN BODIES IN THE RECTUM OR ANUS

1. Do not pull any piece of string that protrudes from the anus. Cut off the excess and confine the animal in a pen or indoors to be sure all the string passes. In many cases one end of a long string catches around the base of the tongue or a tooth and the balance passes all the way through the intestinal tract. Pulling on the string may "shirr" the intestines, like cloth around a pajama string. This would severely injure the intestines, and might even kill the patient. If the string protruding from the anus doesn't pass within a day, take the animal to the veterinarian.

2. Lubricate bone chips and other impacted material with mineral oil (1 teaspoon per 5 pounds of pet). Give once or twice daily in the patient's food; this may help the animal to pass the foreign object.

3. On rare occasions, a sharp object, such as a bone splinter, protrudes from the anus. Remove the object with forceps, using the greatest of care.

Prevention

1. Remember, an infant animal is especially prone to foreign-body problems. Be especially vigilant during the early period of your pet's life. Observe your pet carefully, so that you can remove objects it should not be playing with.

2. Give it only large, strong playthings or bones to chew. This does assist teething. Avoid small, easily torn objects.

3. Once the teething period has passed, train your pet not to mouth or chew things. Good discipline is important for many reasons, and putting an end to the chewing habit is a good way to start training.

9.

Burns and Injuries from Cold (Frostbite, Freezing)

Burns

DEFINITION

A burn is an injury that damages or destroys tissue. It may be caused by heat, electricity, chemicals, or radiation. The seriousness of the burn is greatly compounded by the percentage of the body that is involved. Small or superficial burns are of little concern, while extensive burns may cause death. An extensive burn may kill by shock within the first few hours or by infection within 7 to 10 days.

Superficial burns may just produce a mild increase in blood supply to the area (redness, or inflammation) or destroy the outermost layers of the skin. This may result in peeling (as in sunburn) or loss of hair and temporary minor lesions.

Deeper burns will actually kill the outer layers of the skin and may even "cook" parts of the soft tissue. Without the protective covering of skin, fluids will ooze freely from the body. The loss of fluids produces severe shock, which can be rapidly fatal unless prompt treatment is obtained. Destruction of the skin also leaves the patient vulnerable to invasion by bacteria; infections can develop about a week after the burn, resulting in a serious complication that often leads to death.

An animal trapped in a burning building may suffer minor or severe burns—but in addition, may also inhale hot or poisonous gases, which produce severe respiratory problems.

Heat Burns

CAUSES

Animals don't play with matches, and they are afraid of fire; so burns are quite uncommon in pets. When burns do occur, they are usually the result of an animal being trapped in a burning building or being soaked with a flammable substance that is ignited accidentally or by malicious intent. Because of the extensive and highly flammable hair coat on an animal, burns from flames spread rapidly and are very serious.

One of the most common types of heat burns is that sustained by walking on a hot surface (such as a road, stovetop, or hot roof) or through caustic material. These burns can be either minor or extremely serious. A pet can also be scalded by having hot liquid spilled on it or by being involved in other household accidents.

SIGNS AND SYMPTOMS

Superficial burns, although not particularly serious, are painful to the animal. They redden the skin and may singe the hair, but do not cause it to pull out easily. These burns usually heal rapidly without scarring or complications.

While deep burns are more serious, they may cause less pain, since they may destroy the nerves and thus render them inactive. The deeply burned skin may be white, black, or brown. The hair is gone, or if it remains, it will pull out easily. The patient may be depressed and in shock, especially if large areas are burned. An animal is usually able to recover from even deep burns that involve 15 percent or less of the body surface. However, when more than 50 percent of the body is severely burned, the probability of recovery is very slim, and, for humane reasons, the owner should consider putting the animal to sleep. Any deep burn will require intensive, prolonged care.

Chewing on the cord of a plugged-in electrical appliance can produce a special and serious type of electrical burn. Electrical burns generally occur around the mouth on each side of the lips and there may be a local but red, deeply burned area. Although such burns heal slowly, they are relatively minor. However, the electric shock that accompanies them may cause an irregular heartbeat, which in turn may cause death. Another complication of electrical shock is the accumulation of fluid in the animal's lungs. This condition may develop within a few hours, and it requires intensive veterinary care if the patient is to be saved. (The animal would have rapid, labored breathing, possibly with gurgling sounds or drooling from the mouth.)

FIRST AID FOR HEAT BURNS

PRINCIPLES

    1. Relieve pain.

    2. Prevent or treat shock.

    3. Prevent infection.

    4. Stimulate healing.

PROCEDURES FOR SUPERFICIAL BURNS

    1. Immerse the burned area in cold water (to relieve the pain); then dry gently with a clean towel.

    2. Do not apply butter, grease, or first aid ointments. If the burn is small and you cannot obtain veterinary aid, apply a thin film of antibiotic ointment.

    3. Bandage the area with clean bandages. Apply a thick bandage cover if possible (see pages 166–176). Change bandage daily.

    4. Keep the patient quiet. Seek veterinary advice if the burn appears serious.

PROCEDURES FOR DEEP BURNS

1. Do not apply butter, grease, or first aid ointments.

2. Soak bandage or cloth in cold water and apply it to the burned area.

3. Seek veterinary assistance promptly.

4. When you transport the patient, cover the wet dressing with thick, dry, clean bandages or towels.

5. If there is a delay before obtaining medical help, keep the patient lying down and wrap it in warm blankets.

6. If the patient is conscious and can swallow, give it the following salt solution to drink:

> ½ teaspoon of salt and ½ teaspoon of bicarbonate of soda added to 1 quart of water. Administer in small amounts (1 to 4 ounces at a time, depending on the size of the animal). Repeat in 2 hours if veterinary care has not been obtained. Do not give these fluids if the patient is vomiting.

7. Do not give sedatives, stimulants, or any other drugs without specific veterinary advice.

Chemical Burns

CAUSES

For various reasons, animals come into contact with Mace, acid solutions (toilet-bowl cleaners), or alkalies (drain cleaners). People may throw caustic or petroleum products (kerosene or gasoline) at animals they consider a nuisance or a danger to the environment.

SIGNS AND SYMPTOMS

The animal will feel local pain, especially around the face and eyes. The skin will be red, and there is often an unusual odor about the animal. A caustic substance that has been on the animal for a period of time may have eaten away an area of the skin.

FIRST AID FOR CHEMICAL BURNS

PRINCIPLES

    1. Remove the caustic substance quickly.

    2. Use a soothing ointment or protective substance on the area.

    3. Obtain veterinary care.

PROCEDURES

    1. Wash the area liberally with huge amounts of plain water.

    2. Apply specific antidotes if these are known.

    3. Apply soothing substances such as olive oil, vegetable oil, or antibiotic ointment.

    4. If the eyes are involved, wash the entire face thoroughly and flush the eyes with water. Hold the eyelids open, and with a small bulb syringe, rinse the eyeball well with plain lukewarm water. To be effective, you must do this very soon after the injury and *very thoroughly*.

You cannot expect the animal to cooperate in this procedure. Muzzle and restrain the animal (see pages 151–152 and 159–165) if necessary, as time is of the utmost importance.

    5. If acid has burned the skin, rinse the area well with a solution containing 1 teaspoon of baking soda to 1 quart of water.

    6. If an alkali was involved, rinse with plain water only.

    7. To prevent the animal from scratching the area and making the condition worse, tape the the patient's feet together and/or wrap it in a blanket.

    8. Proceed to a veterinary hospital immediately.

Sunburn

Since most pets have dense hair coats, they are amply shielded from the burning rays of the sun, and so sunburn is essentially unknown in pets. A few breeds of dogs and cats have a "solar skin reaction," characterized by redness and peeling behind the black part of the nose and at the tips of the ears. This is not an emergency problem, but you should have your veterinarian treat it in its early stages.

Injuries from Cold (Frostbite, Freezing)

DEFINITION

Frostbite and freezing are tissue damage caused when crystals form in the fluids of tissues of animals exposed to abnormally low temperatures. Frostbite occurs in local body areas that are poorly protected by the hair coat, such as the tips of the ears, the scrotum, and the foot pads. The injury is accentuated by high winds, high humidity, and the length of time the animal is exposed. The tissue damage produced by freezing is somewhat similar to that caused by burns.

CAUSES AND PREVENTION

Frostbite and freezing usually occur when the animal is left outdoors for a prolonged time in stormy, abnormally cold weather. You can prevent them by keeping a dry, wind-sheltered, straw-lined box as a haven for your pet during these freezing periods. Or—better yet—let the animal stay indoors.

SIGNS AND SYMPTOMS

1. The skin may be pale; it will be painful early in the course but not later. After thawing, the skin may be red and scaly.

2. Severe freezing may cause the skin to peel (cats' ear tips may become rounded and the hairs may regrow white).

FIRST AID FOR INJURIES FROM COLD

PRINCIPLES

1. Rewarm the affected area rapidly.

2. Protect the area from further injury.

3. Treat for shock or respiratory problems as necessary.

PROCEDURES FOR LOCAL FROSTBITE

1. Apply heat, using moist packs or blow dryer, to the affected tissues. The heat should not exceed 102° F. (39° C.). Do not overheat and do not rub or treat the tissues roughly.

2. When the tissues are thawed, apply a thin film of plain vaseline or antiseptic cream.

3. Do not allow the part to refreeze; once damaged, it is more susceptible to frostbite in the future.

PROCEDURES FOR SERIOUS FREEZING

1. An animal that has been severely exposed to cold has a low body temperature and is depressed or even comatose. Restore body heat rapidly by immersing the patient in a bath of warm water (102° - 105° F./39° - 41° C.).

2. After rewarming, feed the animal with a solution of warm milk or water containing ½ teaspoon of salt and ½ teaspoon of baking soda per quart of liquid.

3. Dry the animal gently with towels and a warm blow dryer and wrap it in blankets. Do not rub vigorously, as this may damage the skin excessively.

4. Treat for shock (see pages 39–41).

5. General freezing can cause death. Seek veterinary assistance promptly.

10.

Heatstroke

Definition

Heatstroke is a condition in which an animal collapses because the environmental temperature and humidity have increased beyond the point at which its body-control mechanisms can maintain a normal body temperature.

Causes and Prevention

1. Symptoms develop when an animal has been kept closed up in a car, pen, house, or cement-floored cage without shade, adequate ventilation, or water.

2. Exercise and nervousness accentuate the problem, since they cause the animal to become more heated than normal. If the environment is hot, too, the animal will have even more trouble dissipating the extra heat.

3. Anything that decreases the air flow into and out of the animal's body, decreases the natural cooling process. Dogs and cats with short or "pushed in" noses (such as pugs, bulldogs, and Persian cats) are more prone to heatstroke becase they often have anatomical obstructions in their noses and *throats,* which inhibit a free in-and-out flow of air. The tongue is an important cooling organ in animals. During panting, air is forced back and forth over the tongue. Since the tongue has a rich surface blood supply, the air helps cool the blood quite efficiently. Cats that are heat-stressed drool a great deal and will lick themselves to spread

the saliva on their hair coats. The evaporation of the saliva is an important additional cooling aid.

In addition, young and old animals and animals that have previously experienced heatstroke seem to be especially susceptible to the problem.

4. Remember that the sun moves—a car parked in the shade may soon be in full sunlight. Car windows opened only a few inches *do not* provide adequate ventilation. Never leave animals (or children) unattended in a car parked in a sunny parking lot!

Signs and Symptoms

1. Elevated body temperature (usually above 107° F./41.5° C.).

2. Panting, slobbering from the mouth, vomiting, and diarrhea.

3. Collapse and coma, with hot, dry skin and pale gray lips.

FIRST AID FOR HEATSTROKE

PRINCIPLES

1. Remove animal from the hot environment.

2. Reduce the body temperature.

3. Get to a veterinary hospital promptly—this is a life-threatening emergency.

PROCEDURES

1. Move the animal from the vehicle or enclosure to a cool and shady place.

2. Use a hose to soak the animal with cold water and gently massage the legs and body. Place the patient in front of a fan if possible, to hasten the cooling. Continue this procedure until the animal can be taken to a veterinarian or until the body tempera-

ture is less than 103° F. (39.5° C.). Then gently dry the patient with a towel.

3. If the patient is conscious, allow it to drink small amounts of water. Also, wash its mouth thoroughly with cold water to encourage the cooling process.

4. Give artificial respiration if necessary (see pages 14–16).

5. Get the patient to a veterinary hospital promptly for more comprehensive treatment. If you cannot do so immediately, take the animal's rectal temperature every 15 minutes (see pages 187–189); if the temperature starts to rise again, repeat the cooling process described above.

11.

Chest Injuries

Crushing Injuries

Crushing injuries (see also page 13) are usually caused by automobile accidents, severe falls, or kicks or blows with blunt instruments. The rib may be fractured and the soft tissues severely bruised. The lungs themselves may be bruised or torn (internal wound).

SIGNS AND SYMPTOMS

1. Since this type of chest injury causes great pain with every breath, the animal will attempt to "fix" its ribs so they don't move very much. This restricts the volume of air reaching the lungs.

2. The patient may stand with its legs spread apart, its elbows held away from its chest, and its neck extended.

3. Most of the breathing motions are made with the muscles of the abdomen.

FIRST AID FOR CRUSHING CHEST INJURIES

1. Position the animal so that its head is elevated.

2. Try to place the patient so that the injured side is down. This is often the most comfortable position.

3. Bandage any wounds lightly. Be careful not to restrict breathing.

4. Administer pain-relieving medications for several days. Consult with your veterinarian.

Compression of the Lungs

Following crushing injuries the animal's chest may fill with blood, air, or fluids that will compress the lungs and decrease the volume of air that your pet can breathe in and out. This is an extreme life-threatening emergency!

If your pet develops progressively more labored breathing following even a minor accident, seek veterinary attention immediately!

Penetrating Chest Wounds

Penetrating chest wounds (see also pages 13 and 22–23) are some of the most serious injuries that can befall your pet. You may have only minutes in which to save the patient's life. The greatest danger is that a large wound will let air enter the chest *around* the lungs. The lungs will then collapse, and even though the animal makes breathing motions with its ribs, no air enters the lung passages.

Another grave danger is the possibility that the chest wound will rupture or lacerate the lungs, heart, or one of the great vessels. This may cause fatal hemorrhaging. If the penetrating wound is caused by a sharp instrument and the wounding object is still in place, leave it undisturbed; removing it may cause increased bleeding.

SIGNS AND SYMPTOMS

1. A very deep wound may make a sucking noise as air flows in and out with each breath.

2. There will usually be profuse bleeding from the chest wall or from within the chest.

FIRST AID FOR PENETRATING CHEST WOUNDS

1. Do not muzzle the dog.

2. Prevent air from entering the chest wound by placing a large piece of clean cloth or plastic over the wound and holding it in place with your hand to seal the opening. You must attempt to provide an *airtight* seal; so apply additional padding and bandages to hold your seal in place. However, do not make the bandages so tight that they restrict breathing.

3. If the wounding object is in place, leave it there and incorporate it in the bandages. Support it so it will not move and extend the injury.

4. Treat for shock (see pages 39–41).

5. Place the patient with the injured side down for comfort during transportation.

6. Hurry to a veterinary hospital. Have someone phone ahead to give information about the emergency.

12.

Abdominal Injuries

Deep bruises and penetrating wounds are extremely serious because they usually damage the internal organs. With large wounds, intestines or other organs may protrude from the body and thus be vulnerable to further injury and contamination.

Signs and Symptoms

1. There will be bleeding from lacerations of the abdomen.
2. The abdominal muscles will be very tense.
3. The animal will not want to move around and may be in severe pain.
4. If the wound is large, internal organs may be visible or may even protrude from the wound.
5. The patient may collapse and be in shock (see pages 37–42).

FIRST AID FOR ABDOMINAL WOUNDS

1. Muzzle the dog unless it is vomiting (see page 152).

2. Place sterile or clean dressings over the wound. Moisten the cloth with warm water to help keep the wound and any protruding organs damp.

3. Do not try to replace the organs.

4. Secure the dressings with a firm bandage.

5. Treat for shock (see pages 39–41).

6. Keep the patient level, but if vomiting develops remove the muzzle and be certain the mouth is held so the animal does not inhale the vomitus.

7. Do not give *anything* by mouth because emergency surgery will be necessary.

8. Seek veterinary help immediately.

13.

Eye Injuries

Many breeds of dogs and cats with short snouts, such as pugs, Pekingese, Boston terriers, and Persian cats, have prominently protruding eyes. These animals are particularly susceptible to many types of eye injuries. Foreign objects can be blown or rubbed into the eyes. A dog that rides in a car with its head out the window is especially likely to sustain this type of injury. This habit should never be condoned. Most eye problems are exceedingly painful, and an animal often aggravates the condition severely by scratching and rubbing. Many injuries have the potential of producing permanent ocular defects that involve partial or complete blindness. Prompt restraint and protective care is vital in all eye injuries.

Causes

1. Small particles, such as dust, plant seeds, thorns, twigs, and hair are commonly blown or rubbed into the animal's eye and may become trapped under a lid.

2. Irritants may be sprayed maliciously or accidentally into an animal's face and eyes. Chemicals such as Mace, dog repellents, ammonia, pesticides, shampoos and soaps, orchard sprays, and weed killers may all be hazardous if they come into contact with the eye.

3. Lacerations that involve the eyelid or the eyeball itself can be very serious. Cat scratches commonly cause these injuries. Fishhooks may become lodged in the eyelids. Many eye injuries

occur when the animal investigates an enclosure, such as the inside of a small culvert, box, or can. In such cases the animal startles, rapidly moves its head, and injures its eyes. Automobile accidents and other severe blows may also cut or scratch eyes.

4. Severe blows to the eye usually bruise the surrounding area. Smaller bruises produce closed wounds or hemorrhaging under the skin—the canine or feline equivalent of "black eyes." Because of the animal's hair coat, these are not usually visible.

Signs and Symptoms

1. The eyelids may be closed tightly.
2. There is excessive tearing.
3. The head and eye will be painful; so the animal will resent handling.
4. The eyeball may be red.
5. The animal may paw at the eye or rub the side of the face on the ground.
6. The eye may be swollen and bleeding or the entire eyeball may be pushed forward, so it is completely out of its normal socket (an extreme emergency).

FIRST AID FOR EYE INJURIES

PRINCIPLES

1. Remove the cause.

2. Prevent further injury.

3. Protect the eye from drying.

PROCEDURES

1. Restrain the patient by muzzling or wrapping it in a blanket, so that you can immobilize the head safely and examine the eye carefully.

2. Inspect the eye by gently parting the lids or lifting up on the eyelashes of the upper lid. A bright light is a necessary aid.

3. Rinse the surface of the eyeball and the eyelids with plain water. Apply water with an eye dropper or drip it off a large wad of cotton or tissue. Do not rub the surface of the eye or the eyelid; allow the water to flush the surface of the eyeball. Boric acid is not needed.

4. If you can locate a simple foreign object, remove it with a pledget of moistened cotton or paper tissue. Be very gentle.

5. To obtain a better view of the inner surfaces of the upper lid, place a matchstick horizontally on the outside of the lid. Pull upward on the eyelashes and fold the lid over the matchstick. This will allow you to inspect the undersurface of the lid thoroughly.

6. To control bleeding injuries involving the eyelid, gently apply direct pressure with dry gauze pads. Eye bandages are difficult to keep in place, although strips of adhesive tape may be moderately successful. If you cannot readily control the bleeding, hold the compress gently in place and take the patient to the veterinarian.

7. Bruises involving the eye area usually swell and become red or purple from minor hemorrhages under the skin. Apply cold compresses immediately. (Ice packs may be too cold for applications directly to the eye.)

8. Lacerations of the eyeball itself or foreign objects that penetrate the eyeball are extreme emergencies. Some vision will almost always be lost. If this occurs, place a dampened gauze or cloth compress over the eye and transport the patient to a veterinary hospital at once. Do not attempt to wash the eye or to remove the foreign object. Cover both eyes to help keep the patient quiet.

9. Dogs and cats with large prominent eyes may have an eyeball prolapsed or "popped out" of its socket by blunt injuries or contusions. If the eyeball is out of its socket or if the surface is dry or scratched, it is important to prevent drying. Keep the eye surface moist with drops of "artificial tears," contact-lens solution,

plain water, or cod-liver or olive oil. Apply every 15 to 20 minutes. It may also help to close the lids. These injuries require the prompt attention of a veterinarian who is skilled in animal ophthalmology.

10. Do not attempt first aid for bleeding that occurs inside the eyeball. When this happens, the pupil or the entire eye may appear a vivid red. Take the animal to a veterinarian promptly.

Prevention

1. Do not let your dog ride with its head out the car window.

2. Apply cod-liver oil or ophthalmic ointment to your pet's eyes before bathing or spraying the animal with insecticides.

3. Inspect and cleanse your pet's eyes after it has been running or hunting in heavy grass or brush. Then apply a small amount of protective eye ointment.

4. Do not roughhouse with short-nosed breeds of dogs and cats, and do not grasp them by the neck or restrain them forcibly with tight collars.

5. Inspect your pet's eyes frequently—especially if you notice excessive tearing or pawing at the eyes.

6. Close up any holes in fences, pens, pipes, and boxes, that are small enough to allow a pet to insert only its head and not its body.

14.

Loss of Consciousness

There are several levels of "unconsciousness," ranging from stupor—when the animal is groggy but can be aroused—to complete unresponsiveness.

Causes

Unconsciousness may be due to primary or secondary causes.

Primary causes are those that directly affect the animal's nervous system, such as head injuries (fractures, concussions, etc.); medical diseases, such as tumors, bleeding in the brain, or seizures (fits); or poisonings.

Secondary causes are those in which an injury or disease of some other body system later affects the nervous system. Examples include shock, electric shock, heatstroke, freezing, asphyxia, diabetes, kidney failure, circulatory failure, or cardiac arrest.

Evaluation of an Unconscious Patient

1. *Respiration.* Note whether the respiration is shallow or deep, rapid or slow. Any of these signs may occur in an unconscious patient.

2. *Pupils.* Note whether the pupils of the eye are dilated, whether they are of unequal size, and whether they fail to respond to a bright light by constricting. These are all unfavorable signs.

3. *Blink reflex.* Gently touch the surface of the eye; the animal should blink.

4. *Heart rate.* Take the patient's heart rate by feeling its pulse at the inside of the rear leg (see pages 189–191).

5. *Odor on the breath.* Smell the breath for any unusual odor; try to identify it.

6. *Paralysis.* Determine whether the patient is paralyzed or the muscles are stiff.

7. *Incontinence.* Note whether there is involuntary passage of urine and stool.

Evaluation of Depth of Unconsciousness

1. *Stupor.* The animal is groggy and sleepy but can be aroused if stimulated. Its pupils respond to light and it blinks when the cornea is touched.

2. *Coma.* In this, a deeper state of unconsciousness, the patient cannot be aroused, the pupils do not respond to light, and the blink reflex is gone. The patient will not feel pain if its feet are pinched very hard. Breathing may be slow and shallow, and the pulse may be weak and hard to count.

Determination of Death

Do not assume that an animal is dead merely because obvious signs of life are absent. The following, listed in order of occurrence after death, are reliable indications of death.

1. *Cessation of breathing.* Hold a wisp of cotton near the nose and look for movement or hold a mirror at the nose and look for fogging.

2. *Absence of heartbeat.* Take the pulse at the rear leg (see page 189) or feel the chest just behind the elbow (see pages 190–191).

3. *Eye changes.* The pupils become widely dilated and do not respond to light. The surface of the eyeball becomes dull and dry, and the eyeball loses its firmness.

4. *Incontinence.* Urine and sometimes feces may be passed spontaneously.

5. *Drop in body temperature.* The body temperature falls over a period of an hour, so that the feet feel cool. The rectal temperature is below 80° F. (27° C.).

6. *Changes in muscle tone.* The muscles become very flaccid and soft at the time of death; later rigor mortis sets in, and the muscles then become stiff. As decay begins, the muscles soften again and the body develops an unpleasant odor.

FIRST AID FOR UNCONSCIOUSNESS

1. Treat for shock (see pages 39–41).

2. Do not give anything by mouth.

3. Obtain veterinary assistance at once! The emergency is of the utmost urgency.

15.

Convulsions (Seizures or Fits)

Definition

A convulsion is a temporary but sudden loss of consciousness accompanied by severe involuntary contractions of the skeletal muscles. The condition is usually associated with drooling huge quantities of saliva from the mouth and with involuntary urination. Although seizures are disturbing to both the animal and its owner, they seldom last more than one minute, after which they spontaneously lessen and stop. Depending on the cause, they may recur at regular or at infrequent intervals. In rare instances, a seizure may continue for several hours. This is the most serious type of seizure, and it may cause death. Prompt veterinary care is essential in such a case.

The brief convulsion will usually stop long before the patient can be transported to a veterinary hospital and will rarely cause death. After one of these brief seizures you should schedule a nonemergency veterinary examination to determine the cause of the problem and the course to follow for future medical care.

Causes

Convulsions range from simple to very serious problems and are caused by a variety of conditions. In some cases the exact cause cannot be determined. Some specific causes are listed below.

1. Infectious diseases due to viral, fungal, or bacterial agents; tetanus.

2. Tumors of the brain or pancreas.

3. Severe head injuries (as sustained in automobile accidents).

4. Overheating or high fever.

5. Drugs or poisons (lead, insecticides, etc.).

6. Metabolic abnormalities: low blood sugar, or low calcium (as after whelping), urinary diseases, etc.

7. Parasites (only in very young animals).

8. Inherited or congenital defects (such as hydrocephalus, or "water on the brain").

9. Idiopathic—that is, "of unknown cause." This is true of a high percentage of seizures in all animals, including man. More research is needed to determine why seizures occur.

Signs and Symptoms

1. There is a sudden onset of apprehension, restlessness, whining, and minor muscle twitching (often around the face and lips). This is followed closely by complete collapse and loss of consciousness.

2. The animal falls onto its side and is racked by spastic and violent contractions of all the skeletal muscles.

3. The mouth may open and close rapidly and the animal drools profusely. The patient may also pass urine spontaneously.

4. After a very few moments the spasms become less severe and the patient rests—breathing heavily.

5. Sudden noises or abrupt handling may increase the spasms or precipitate another convulsion.

6. The patient is often wobbly and dazed for a time after recovery and is usually quite hungry.

7. Cats that are having a convulsion may also show rage or become hysterical in addition to the above symptoms.

FIRST AID FOR CONVULSIONS

PRINCIPLES

1. Prevent injury to patient or bystanders.

2. Do not give medications, place objects in the mouth, or apply excessive restraint.

3. Give artificial respiration if breathing stops.

4. If seizures continue for 5 to 10 minutes, seek veterinary care immediately. Usually the seizure will be brief. In this case, have your veterinarian examine the animal at a convenient time.

PROCEDURES

1. Prevent injury by protecting the patient so that it doesn't do such things as fall down stairs, stagger into a road, or fall into a pond.

2. Mildly restrain the patient by confining it with a blanket, but keep your hands away from its mouth. Do not muzzle the patient, give it any medication, or place anything between its teeth.

3. An animal in a seizure, typically, is not aggressive or vicious, but since it can't control its jaw muscles, it may damage anything placed in its mouth (even the fingers of a beloved owner). If there is any doubt, shut the animal in a room and leave it alone for 10 minutes.

4. If breathing stops, give artificial respiration (see pages 14–16).

5. Be prepared to give the veterinarian all relevant information when you present the patient for a later (nonemergency) physical examination.

    a. Dates, description, and duration of previous seizures.

    b. All medications and drugs the animal is currently receiving.

c. Any exposure to poisons, any strange materials the animal may have chewed on or eaten.

d. The patient's family history of seizures and diseases.

e. Any recent personality changes.

f. Any recent changes in the eating, sleeping, urinary, or bowel-movement patterns.

g. The animal's vaccination history.

h. Recent contact with other animals.

i. Previous illness or injuries, with dates of each.

j. A description of your animal's seizure episode, with emphasis on the length and timing and on how the animal acted before and after the seizure.

Prevention

Prevention is difficult because seizures have many known causes—and many unknown ones. There is still much to learn about this problem. However, the following precautions will be helpful.

1. Keep vaccinations up-to-date for distemper, hepatitis, parainfluenza, and rabies.

2. Have regular veterinary examinations.

3. Feed an "ideal" balanced diet to your pet (see pages 203–209).

4. Protect your pet from injury or poisoning by keeping it leashed or confined and under control at all times.

5. Use only drugs prescribed or approved by your veterinarian.

6. If your pet has epilepsy (idiopathic convulsions), don't despair—many epileptic animals live long, happy lives, with infrequent or completely controlled seizures.

7. Work with your veterinarian to pinpoint the cause if possible.

8. Follow prescriptions explicitly. Regular medication is an ab-

solute must. You should continue it whether or not your pet is having seizures, since the drug effect is cumulative and often produces its best results only after prolonged dosage. Some patients respond much better to one medication than to another; other patients will need a combination of anticonvulsant drugs. This is a matter of individual response; so your pet's veterinarian may need to arrive at the best medication regimen by trial and error over a period of time. It is necessary to tailor a plan to your pet's special problem. Be patient, cooperative, and understanding.

9. In spite of expert care, a few epileptic patients may have an occasional mild seizure. In almost all of these cases the problem is tolerable because of the long intervals of normal behavior between seizures. In some instances, however, control is not possible (conditions caused by brain tumor, some poisons, and some viral or fungal infections).

16.

Head Injuries

Lacerations

Head wounds tend to bleed profusely, since the head is richly supplied with blood. These wounds may also damage many important nerves and blood vessels. Deep lacerations may injure the eye or ear, and may even penetrate the skull, injuring the brain.

FIRST AID FOR HEAD INJURIES

1. Do not attempt to cleanse the wound.

2. Apply a sterile dressing and use *gentle* pressure to control bleeding. If there is a fracture, excessive pressure may force sharp bone fragments into the brain or other vital structures, thus producing additonal serious injury.

3. Apply a bandage to hold the dressing in place.

4. Seek veterinary help promptly.

Brain Injuries

Open or closed wounds caused by a blow from a blunt instrument, an automobile accident, or a fall from a cliff or a fire escape may produce brain damage (lacerations or concussions).

SIGNS AND SYMPTOMS

1. Loss of consciousness. Progressive deepening of coma is an unfavorable sign.

2. Bleeding or escape of clear fluid from the ears, nose, or mouth.

3. Vomiting.

4. Pupils are different sizes.

5. Signs of general shock (pages 38–39).

6. Paralysis, especially of one side of the body; loss of control of bowel or bladder.

FIRST AID FOR BRAIN INJURIES

1. Keep the patient lying down, flat on its side.

2. Maintain an open airway.

3. Give artificial respiration if necessary (see pages 14–16).

4. Treat for shock (see pages 39–41).

5. Gently bandage to control bleeding.

6. Do not give anything by mouth.

7. Get the patient to a veterinary hospital promptly.

Face, Nose, and Jaw Injuries

Wounds and fractures in the facial region may damage vital structures, but this danger is compounded by the swelling and bleeding, which may obstruct the patient's airway.

Nosebleeds in animals are commonly caused by foreign objects in the nostrils and by blows to the nose. In rare cases they are caused by general bleeding disorders.

You can readily stop the common nosebleed with simple treatment.

FIRST AID FOR FACE, NOSE, AND JAW INJURIES

1. For nosebleeds, place cold compresses on the top and sides of the nose and apply pressure. You may moisten gauze strips and place them into the nasal opening, but this is a small area and the patient will not usually cooperate. If the bleeding recurs, ask your veterinarian to examine your pet.

2. For extensive face and jaw injuries, treat unconsciousness (if necessary) and shock.

   a. Lower the animal's face so that the blood and fluids can drain away from the throat.

   b. Clear the airway. Pull the tongue forward and remove any foreign material in the mouth (see pages 70–72).

   c. Give artificial respiration if necessary (see pages 14–16).

   d. Treat for shock (see pages 39–41).

   e. Try to control bleeding (see pages 23–28).

   f. If you must move the patient, do so with great caution, since injuries to the face are often complicated by head and neck injuries. Careless movements may seriously increase the original damage. Support the head and neck so they don't "flop around."

Ear Injuries

Animals rarely show signs of a ruptured ear drum, and although it may occur, it often heals spontaneously. However, dogs and cats commonly lacerate the ears. This may result from fights (raccoons, cats, or dogs), from entanglement in barbed wire or thorns, or from self-mutilation due to severe itching. Hunting dogs are especially prone to ear injuries.

The ear has a very rich blood supply, and so injuries result in profuse bleeding. Severe head shaking or scratching may rupture a vein in the ear flap and cause a large, soft swelling of the ear. This "blood blister" will need veterinary treatment, but it is not an emergency. Severe ear infections caused by bacteria or small parasites called ear mites may cause the shaking. These infections must be treated to remove the cause of the head shaking.

FIRST AID FOR EAR INJURIES

1. Stop the bleeding by applying direct pressure to the wound with sterile gauze.

2. Dress and bandage the wound. To do this, lay the ear flat over the top of the head, cover it on both sides with gauze pads, lay cotton on top, and bandage it firmly in place. It is important to do this to immobilize the ear, or else bleeding will soon start again.

3. Take your pet to a veterinary hospital if the injury is severe. An extensive cut needs suturing and special care. If the laceration is small, you can often treat it well at home (see pages 21–34).

Prevention of Head Injuries

1. Control your pet by discipline, leashing, or confinement.
2. Do not allow it access to fire escapes, roofs, areas with open windows, or play areas adjacent to any sort of precipice (gorge, cliff).
3. Certain types of hunting dogs will inevitably have fights with other animals, but here again, training and good control will minimize injury.

17.

Spinal Injuries

Causes

Injuries to the spinal cord most commonly result from a severe blow or an accident, such as an automobile crash, that causes fractures or bleeding. However, many dogs develop bone disease, tumors, disc problems, and other slow-developing conditions. Eventually the disease process reaches a stage where even mild stress or light exercise (jumping off furniture or climbing stairs) causes damage to the spinal cord, and the dog becomes wobbly, paralyzed, or otherwise incapacitated.

Signs and Symptoms

1. Symptoms develop suddenly, often shortly after an accident.
2. There may be a wobbly gait.
3. There may be paralysis of one or more legs. Sometimes the legs are straightened out stiffly.
4. Bruising and swelling may occur in a region of the neck or spine. In the neck region this may cause difficulty in breathing.
5. The patient may not feel pain when you pinch its feet or legs.
6. There may be paralysis or impairment of normal urination and defecation.

FIRST AID FOR SPINAL INJURIES

1. Do not alter the patient's position.

2. Make sure breathing is not impaired. Clear the airway (see pages 14 and 70–71) and give artificial respiration if necessary (see pages 14–16).

3. Bandage any wounds of the neck or back to control bleeding and prevent contamination (see pages 169–176).

4. Get the patient to a veterinary hospital promptly since delay of more than a few hours may decrease the possibility of successful treatment. You must be *extremely* careful when you move the animal. Use the following procedures:

   a. Do not bend the neck or allow the backbone to jackknife or bend in abnormal positions.

   b. *Slide* the patient onto a board or blanket by pulling the legs carefully in a direction perpendicular to the spine. With a small dog, grasp the loose skin on the neck *and* back and slide the patient, back first, onto the board. If you use a blanket, pull it onto something solid so the patient will not sag when lifted. This method works well for fairly large dogs.

   c. Load cats and smaller dogs into a solid, appropriate-sized cardboard box for safe transportation. Break down one side of the box so that you can slide the patient in smoothly. Then tape or tie the side of the box in its original position. This system provides a safe and comfortable carrier.

18.

Leg Injuries

In addition to lacerations (see page 22), leg injuries from major accidents include damage to the bones, joints, ligaments, tendons, and adjacent soft tissues.

Definitions

FRACTURE

A fracture is a break or crack in a bone.

A greenstick fracture is a crack (an incomplete break) in a bone without displacement of the bone.

A simple fracture is a complete break in a bone that does not pierce the skin. There will, however, always be extensive soft-tissue damage in the fracture area.

A compound fracture is a complete break in a bone that does pierce the skin. These injuries are very serious since contamination is present and infection may follow. Simple fractures may become compound ones if you do not handle them properly, since the sharp ends of the fractured bones can easily puncture the surrounding skin.

A comminuted fracture is a series of complete breaks that chip, splinter, or fragment the bone. It may be simple or compound.

DISLOCATION

A dislocation is the displacement of bones from a joint, which results from injury to the supporting soft tissues or the joint capsule. A dislocation may be associated with a fracture, in which case the fracture involves the joint surface. Such an injury is serious, as it usually causes permanently impaired joint mobility.

SPRAIN

A sprain is a stretching or tearing of the tendons or ligaments supporting a joint. It is associated with bruising and swelling of soft tissues around the joint, but there is no dislocation or fracture.

STRAIN

A strain is a stretching or tearing of a muscle, which is often associated with sprains, dislocations, or fractures.

Fractures

CAUSES

Most fractures in pet animals are caused by automobile accidents or falls from great heights. Fractures either result from direct force applied to the site of the break or from indirect force applied at some distance from the break (as when a dog jumps out of a window and lands on its feet but breaks a bone in the leg). In some cases improperly balanced diets (all meat), cancer of the bone, or other diseases weaken the bones so that relatively trivial injuries produce fractures.

SIGNS AND SYMPTOMS

1. Sudden onset of acute pain in a local area of the leg.
2. Local swelling.
3. Deformity of leg structure. Often there will be a marked difference in the size, shape, and length of the leg; this is especially evident in comparison to its normal counterpart on the other side of the body.

4. Grating sounds of bones rubbing together with even slight movement.

5. Loss of function or of motion. Often the leg will just hang limply, unable to support weight.

FIRST AID FOR FRACTURES

PRINCIPLES

1. Immobilize the fracture so the ends of the fractured bones do not produce more injury and pain.

2. Treat for shock.

3. Treat associated wounds and other injuries.

4. Transport the patient promptly and safely to a veterinary hospital.

5. Do not attempt to set a fracture or touch a bone that protrudes from a deep wound.

PROCEDURES

1. Muzzle the patient (see page 152), since it will be in severe pain and will resent handling.

2. Keep the patient on its side with the injured leg uppermost.

3. Grasp the animal by the skin at the scruff of the neck and by a fold of skin over the hips and pull it, back first, onto a blanket or board. Use this as a sled to slide the patient out of traffic or any other dangerous area. If nothing is available for a sled, slide the animal carefully along the ground, allowing its legs to follow along in a straight line. This will not place any angular or distorting forces on the injured leg.

4. Give artificial respiration (pages 14–16) and treat for bleeding (see pages 23–28) if necessary.

5. Do not replace exposed bone fragments—but cover them with a gauze dressing and a light bandage (see pages 167–174) to protect them from further contamination.

6. Treat for shock (see pages 39–41).

7. Prevent motion of the injured leg and its joints.

8. Apply an improvised splint so the patient can be transported safely (see below).

9. Get to a veterinary hospital promptly. Position the animal with the injured part up during the trip.

SPLINTING

1. It is more difficult to apply temporary splints to pet animals than it is to people because the legs of dogs and cats are more tapered and angular in conformation, especially at the upper parts, close to the body. Splints are thus most practical for fractures involving the lower, straighter part of the legs.

2. Always splint or otherwise immobilize an injured leg if there is any suspicion of a fracture. Splinting is also desirable for such injuries as dislocations and sprains.

3. Improvise a splint from handy materials. Folded newspapers, magazines, cardboard strips, or towels will give good support. Narrow pieces of board, straight sticks, folded wire hardware cloth, and screening are also useful.

4. *Making a splint:*

    a. The splint should be long enough to include and extend beyond the joints at either end of the fractured bone.

    b. Use padding between the splint and the skin, especially over the joint areas. (If you make the splint of folded towels, you do not need padding.)

    c. If you make your splint of wood or some other inflexible material, use two separate parts: one for the outside

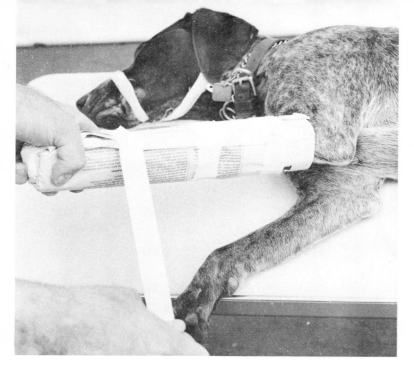

FIGURE 9. *A temporary splint.* Wrap a folded newspaper around the injured leg and tape it firmly in place. It may slide off, but it will serve well enough for a short trip to the hospital.

surface of the leg and the other for the inside surface. Fold a splint made from newspapers, magazines, towels, or "hardware" cloth into a U-shaped "trough" and place the leg into the trough (see Figure 9).

Dislocations

CAUSES

Most dislocations occur as a result of severe falls, blows, or automobile accidents. Once the soft tissues supporting a joint are injured enough to allow a dislocation, the chances of repeated dislocation are greatly enhanced.

111

SIGNS AND SYMPTOMS

1. Acute pain in the joint.

2. Swelling and deformity of the joint area and length of the leg in contrast to its counterpart on the opposite side of the body.

3. Pain on motion of or pressure on the joint.

4. Limited movement or immobility of the joint.

FIRST AID FOR DISLOCATIONS

1. Use the same general procedures described in "First Aid for Fractures" (see pages 109–111).

2. Immobilize the affected joint in a splint or heavily padded bandage.

3. Do not attempt to correct the deformity of the joint, as you may cause further injury.

4. Seek veterinary aid.

Sprains

CAUSES

Sprains are often caused by lesser forces than those producing fractures or dislocations. The force moves a limb beyond its joint's normal range of motion and this stretches and tears tendons, ligaments, and other soft tissue structures around the joint. Sprains are less common in animals than in people. These injuries are easily confused with dislocations or simple fractures; so X-ray examination is usually desirable.

SIGNS AND SYMPTOMS

1. Swelling.

2. Pain on touching or moving the joint.

3. Limited use of the joint (possibly).

FIRST AID FOR SPRAINS

1. Rest the part by splinting if necessary (see pages 110–111).

2. Apply cold packs in the first few hours after the injury. Put crushed ice into a plastic bag, wrap the bag in a towel, and apply the pack to the swollen joint for 10 to 15 minutes every 2 hours.

3. If there is no relief of pain and swelling after several days, seek veterinary advice.

Strains

CAUSES

Torn muscles may occur with other injuries, but they often result from severe overexertion, especially of muscles that are in poor condition. Animals such as racing greyhounds and hunting dogs that have not been properly warmed up prior to sudden physical exertion are particularly prone to muscle strains.

SIGNS AND SYMPTOMS

1. Sudden lameness.

2. Tension or "knotting" of a group of muscles.

3. Pain and swelling in the area.

FIRST AID FOR STRAINS

1. Treat early injuries as for sprains—with cold packs and rest.

2. After the first day continue rest but change to moist-heat applications. Wrap moist towels around the affected leg for 15 minutes every 2 hours during the day.

3. Seek veterinary advice if, after several days, there is no relief of pain and lameness.

Prevention of Leg Injuries

1. Automobile accidents are the single greatest cause of leg injuries in pets. Communities with leash laws have many fewer injuries to their pets. It is of prime importance to keep your pet leashed, penned, or confined to your property and under your direct control. Do not allow pets to ride in the rear of a truck or to lean out of the window of a moving vehicle.

2. Do not allow pets to play on a roof garden, balcony, or fire escape; near a cliff or river gorge; or in any other place where a fall can occur.

3. Keep your pet away from operating machinery, such as tractors and mowers.

4. Keep your pet's toenails clipped short so they will not catch in rugs or other floor or ground coverings and precipitate a fall.

5. Do not leave your pet unattended on a table or in a bathtub during a treatment, grooming, or bathing procedure. The animal may jump off or out and severely injure a leg.

6. If you are going to exercise the animal strenuously, as in hunting or racing, get it into proper physical condition by gradually increasing the amount of exercise on a daily basis. Prior to each workout, warm the animal up gradually, to get its muscles supple, well supplied with blood, and ready for the extreme exertion.

When the exercise is over, cool the animal out—that is, keep it walking for a few minutes.

19.

Urinary Problems

There are three urgent problems of the urinary tract that require prompt care: urinary obstruction, rupture of the bladder, and blood in the urine.

Urinary Obstruction

Urinary obstruction is common in male cats, less common in male dogs, and rare in female dogs or cats. The male urinary passage (urethra) is long and narrow, which allows crystals and stones to become compacted and thus dam-up the passageway in the penis. The female urethra is short and wider and will easily pass many of the stones.

There are many kinds of urinary stones. Some are caused by infection or by inherited metabolic defects; an improper diet may accentuate the problem once it has started. Control and prevention is complex and not always successful. The treatment objective is to promote a large production of dilute urine. This may be achieved through special diet or medication. Treatment varies with the individual patient.

When the urinary tract is completely obstructed, the animal will not be able to urinate and will strain to do so. Sometimes a few drops of urine will pass. A cat will sit in its litter box to strain and may appear constipated. Feel the rear of the cat's abdomen. That tense organ (it may feel like a tennis ball) is the distended bladder. It is essential that the cat receive prompt veterinary care.

The patient will be most uncomfortable and will die within 48 to 72 hours if relief is not obtained.

The position for urination the dog assumes is more typical than that of the cat. You can, therefore, easily recognize a dog with a urinary problem. Feel a dog's abdomen in the same way as you would a cat's; the dog's bladder will also be distended. Professional care to catheterize the bladder and relieve the obstruction is mandatory.

Rupture of the Bladder

The bladder may rupture if the pet receives a severe blow in the abdomen (such as being hit by a car) when the bladder is distended. It is imperative to observe the animal for passage of urine. Abdominal pain, failure to urinate, and sudden depression and distention of the abdomen are signs that may indicate the bladder is ruptured. Without surgical repair, a ruptured bladder can cause death in 2 to 3 days.

Blood in the Urine

Although in some cases it is mild, blood in the urine is always a sign of trouble. An animal that has sustained a severe injury, such as being hit by a car, may have a severe closed wound (see pages 33–34) of the kidney, bladder, or tubular urinary passageways. Bleeding may be severe enough to cause shock and possible death. The absence of urine, or the presence of bloody urine following an accident indicate an extreme emergency. Obtain veterinary aid immediately.

Chronic bloody urination, with smaller or sporadic discharge of blood, may result from a urinary infection, tumor, or from the irritation rough stones produce in the urinary system. The blood will persist until the malady is properly treated. These problems require prompt, but not emergency, veterinary care.

20.

Reproductive Problems

This section is written to describe normal reproductive processes, with brief comments about problems which may arise. Methods are outlined for handling the common problems.

Reproductive Problems of Dogs

The breeding cycle in a bitch lasts for approximately 6 months, and the female is "in season" for approximately 21 days at the beginning of the cycle. The cycle starts (puberty) when the bitch is 7 to 12 months of age. Each "season" is characterized by swollen external genitalia and a bloody discharge that turns to a yellowish color and becomes thicker after about 10 days. Ovulation occurs after this time, and the female will accept breeding for only about 7 to 10 days during this period. The copious bloody discharge is of no health concern, but it is messy and it does attract male dogs, which is a decided nuisance. The congregation of males will loiter about the bitch's home quarters, bark and howl, and often fight among themselves. The female is restless, too, and is quite clever at escaping confinement. It is not wise, of course, to tie the female outside or even to pen her up. She may escape, or a male may gain entrance to the pen. It is best to confine the bitch indoors or to board her in a secure kennel facility for 3 weeks when you notice the first tinges of the bloody vulval discharge.

BREEDING

On or about the 12th day after the vulval discharge first appears, the bitch is ready to accept breeding. If you want your pet to conceive, you should breed her at least 3 times, at 48-hour intervals. Keep the breeding pair separated until this time and allow them to come together only while each is restrained by a collar and leash. If they fight or snap, you can easily pull them apart. The female will indicate her readiness for breeding by standing quietly. The male will mount and copulate for several minutes. After breeding, the male and female genitalia swell and "lock together" for about 30 minutes, a normal condition that dog breeders call a tie. The pair cannot be separated during this time. They will usually stand back to back, but facing in opposite directions. When the tie has relaxed, they will separate spontaneously. During the tie, hold the dogs together, as forceful pulling by either animal may cause injury to the genitalia.

Occasionally, the male's penis does not retract into its protective sheath after breeding. This condition will dry or damage the delicate membranes if it persists. Should this occur, coat the penis with vegetable oil and use gentle manipulation to correct the problem. If the penis has not retracted into the sheath after about an hour, you should get veterinary advice.

MISALLIANCE (MISMATING)

If breeding takes place against your wishes, there is no immediate action you can take. Wait for the tie to release. (Dousing the pair with water or using physical abuse is ineffective in hastening the separation—and it is cruel.) If you take the female to the veterinarian within 48 hours after breeding, hormonal treatment will usually prevent pregnancy (douching is completely ineffective). After treatment, keep the bitch properly confined through the balance of her season so she will not breed again.

PREGNANCY

The normal length of pregnancy is 63 days (see the gestation table on page 259), but a few days' variation is usual. However, pups born more than one week early rarely survive. Natural abortions may occur early in pregnancy and go unobserved by the owner, since the bitch will often eat her pups and lick away any genital discharge.

The newly conceived puppies do not become attached to the lining of the uterus (womb) until about 3 weeks after breeding. The first 3 weeks are a critical time since illness, worm remedies, or some medications given at that time may disturb the pregnancy and even cause death of the pups. Pregnancy can be diagnosed with a high degree of accuracy by feeling the enlarged uterus in the bitch's abdomen between 25 and 30 days after breeding.

As pregnancy advances, the nipples enlarge, the abdomen distends, and at about 42 days, the breasts enlarge. A few days before whelping (giving birth), milk will appear in the breasts. A day or so before whelping the bitch may seek seclusion and tear up papers or cloths to make a nest; she will abruptly reduce her food intake.

On occasion a bitch will experience a "false pregnancy," in which she shows all the above signs but is not pregnant. This condition is caused by a hormonal imbalance, and you may need to have a veterinarian examine or X-ray her to be certain there are no puppies. In time the bitch returns to normal, but for a week or two she may try to "mother" dolls or pieces of cloth and otherwise act strangely. There is no treatment except reducing the food intake and encouraging abundant exercise to reduce the milk in the breasts.

Feeding and exercise are especially important during pregnancy. The bitch should be exercised daily—but not strenuously—to keep her in optimum physical condition. Often an owner allows a pregnant bitch to get too soft and fat. Do not pamper yours! If the bitch is not obese, you can feed her the regular maintenance diet at the same rate per pound as before breeding. When she begins to gain weight due to the growth of her puppies (usually at 35 days), her food should be increased proportionately. Thus, it is necessary to weigh her each week. During the last 28 days of pregnancy, supplement her diet with cottage cheese, cooked eggs, or fresh liver. These protein sources are desirable in all cases. However, vitamin and mineral supplements are rarely necessary for normal bitches receiving a complete, balanced commercial diet. If there is any question in your mind about your pet's diet, get advice from your veterinarian.

As the pregnancy progresses, the puppies in the womb take up more room in the abdomen and leave less room for the bitch's stomach to expand with food. Concurrently, the bitch will need more food, so it is desirable to divide her daily ration into 3 or 4 meals.

Be certain the bitch does not become constipated—especially near term—as this may cause difficulty in whelping. Mineral oil or Colace, given orally, are helpful in regulating the stools. An enema may be needed in some instances.

WHELPING PREPARATIONS

Three weeks before whelping, provide a box so that the bitch will become accustomed to it and feel secure there. It should be large enough for her to stretch out comfortably and still leave room for the pups. It should have sides that are high enough to keep the puppies in and the drafts out, but low enough to allow the bitch to enter and leave easily. Line the box with many thicknesses of newspapers for bedding and for easy cleaning. Attach a bumper rail, about 2 inches by 2 inches, along the sides 2 inches above the floor of the box. This will help keep the puppies from being crowded or smothered by their mother.

Put the box in a warm, quiet room and suspend an infrared bulb just above it (about 3 feet from floor) to provide an accessory heat source. Since chilling is a major cause of puppy deaths, you should use the heat bulb to keep a large area of the whelping box at a temperature of 80° to 85° F. (27° to 29° C.). This will allow the mother and pups to choose a warmer or cooler spot as necessary. The location you choose for the whelping area should be isolated enough to provide a quiet, peaceful environment—but convenient enough to enable you to peek in and keep track of progress without disturbing the new family.

SIGNS OF LABOR

1. The bitch will make a nest 2 or 3 days before whelping.

2. At about the same time, the breasts enlarge and milk appears.

3 The external genitalia become enlarged, soft, and flabby.

4. Often food will be refused just a day before whelping.

5. Twenty-four hours before whelping, the bitch's temperature will drop approximately 2° F. (1° C.). This is a very reliable sign—so if you wish to estimate the whelping time, take the bitch's temperature twice daily and record it on a chart. When you observe the temperature drop, you will know that the puppies are due within 24 hours.

6. A thick mucous discharge appears. This is soon followed by a thin greenish discharge, which indicates that pups should appear within a few hours.

7. During early or primary labor, uterine contractions make the bitch restless. She will not show pain, however.

8. During actual, or secondary, labor, the bitch will noticeably strain with her abdominal muscles and actively expel puppies. Pups should appear within 6 hours after labor starts. If they do not, veterinary assistance is essential.

DELIVERY OF PUPPIES

Pups may be born head first or tail first, and they may or may not be wrapped in a membrane. All these occurrences are normal. But if the membrane covers the head, you must strip it away immediately—but carefully—so the puppy can breathe. If the pup is only partially expelled, you may gently grasp the presenting part and carefully pull out and down, toward the mother's feet. The pups are slippery; so use a soft, clean cloth to get a better grip. As the bitch strains, pull gently and then hold firmly as she relaxes. When she strains again, repeat.

Do not use undue force—and do not insert *anything* into the birth canal. Keep everything you handle clean, and if delivery is not easy, call your veterinarian for advice.

Pups are usually delivered at 30-to-60-minute intervals, but variations are common. If longer periods between births persist, it may be necessary to have veterinary help.

If the placenta does not separate spontaneously, tear the umbilical cord apart between your fingers at a point about 2 inches from the abdomen of the puppy.

As you deliver each pup, present it to the mother so she can clean, warm, and mother it properly. *Do not disturb* when all is going well, as it is important for the pup to nurse soon after delivery. Almost all bitches will complete whelping better if left in peace and seclusion.

WEAK PUPPIES

If a delivered pup appears weak or lifeless and is being ignored by the bitch, you may be able to revive it. These pups are cold, blue, and limp, and they breathe spasmodically—or perhaps not at all. In such cases:

1. Clear membranes and fluids from the nose and mouth.

2. Hold the pup firmly and swing it, head down, several times to help drain fluid from its chest and throat.

3. Fold the pup in a rough, warm towel and rub and pat it briskly. Be fairly rough, as you want to stimulate breathing.

4. If there is no breathing response, blow *gently* into the puppy's mouth or gently compress its chest with your fingers to produce artificial respiration (see pages 14–16). If this fails, the shock of dipping it into alternate pans of warm and cool water may help. Be sure to dry it thoroughly. As soon as the pup is breathing on its own, allow the bitch to take over the mothering and stimulating process of licking and massage.

AFTER WHELPING

Signs that the last pup has been delivered:

1. The bitch is calm and relaxed and is mothering the pups well.

2. She is not straining.

3. Her abdomen is empty and you cannot feel pups when you press your fingers deeply into her flanks.

4. Veterinary examination, including X-rays, may be necessary to be sure—especially in large breeds. Be sure, not sorry! An injection to help shrink the uterus at this time is highly recommended.

Take the bitch out frequently to relieve herself. Use these opportunities to clean the whelping box and examine the puppies. Any deformed pups (harelip, cleft palate, or deformed legs) should be disposed of during the first 24 hours.

After natural whelping most bitches will lick and clean the puppies thoroughly and in the process ingest the placental membranes. This material may upset her digestive system and produce a dark-colored diarrhea. Give a single dose of milk of magnesia (see page 253) to help resolve the problem.

Later, in the course of normal nursing, the puppies' teeth grow in and their toenails become sharp. You should clip the nails to help prevent their scratching the mother's breasts and nipples. But as the teeth become sharp, she will rapidly initiate the weaning process herself.

If the pup's nursing causes the breasts to become irritated, cover one or two nipples with a binder to shift the pup's attention to other nipples. Apply cod-liver oil ointment to the irritated nipples before covering them. This will aid healing and help keep them soft.

UTERINE INFECTION

The genital discharge of the bitch will be dark or bloody for a few hours after whelping but will then normally change to a brownish mucoid material, which may persist for 2 weeks. As the uterus contracts, the material is discharged in a natural cleansing process. If the discharge increases in volume and/or becomes watery, red, and foul-smelling, this is an indication of an infection called metritis. When this happens, the bitch will strain, refuse food, act depressed, and have a fever above 104° F. (40° C.). This is an illness that demands *immediate* veterinary care. Remove the puppies from their mother and feed them formula (see pages 126–128 and 260–261) until the infection is under control.

ECLAMPSIA

During the first month of lactation (nursing the puppies), the mother supplies all the puppies' nutrition through her milk. Their demands may be so great that she develops a blood calcium deficiency called eclampsia. Although it is a rare disorder, it may be seen in small, nervous breeds (Chihuahuas, toy poodles, beagles) and especially in those bitches that have a large number of fat puppies—indicating an abundant milk supply. It is virtually impossible to prevent this rare disorder, but it can be treated satisfactorily if calcium injections are given early in the disease. *This is a real emergency—and delay of treatment for even a few hours may be fatal.*

SIGNS AND SYMPTOMS

1. Onset usually 1 to 4 weeks after whelping.
2. Restlessness, nervousness, and panting.
3. Muscular incoordination and staggering.
4. Excessive drooling.
5. Actual seizures or trembling and shaking muscles.

Take this pet to your veterinarian immediately—even if it is the middle of the night!

MASTITIS

Occasionally, a single breast will become very hard (caked), turn red or purple, and be very painful. This is an infection called mastitis. Since the bitch develops a fever and becomes very sick, remove the pups for hand feeding. Take the bitch to a veterinarian for treatment of the infection.

FEEDING THE LACTATING BITCH AND THE PUPPIES

After whelping, give the bitch broth or milk and a light gruel of regular food several times daily. After the first day, her appetite will rapidly improve, and if she has a large litter, she may be eating three times her normal amount of food by the tenth day. Feed her at least three times daily. Supplement the diet with milk, liver, and eggs—all good for milk supply.

Puppies should gain weight every day after they are born; a level weight or a weight *loss* is a very serious problem. A puppy will double its birth weight by the time it is 14 days old—and since all its food comes from the mother's milk, don't skimp when feeding the bitch. It is wise to offer the puppies a gruel when they are about 16 to 20 days of age and are beginning to crawl around and explore their environment. Make the gruel of milk and soft-moist dog food; this is excellent for puppies. It should be very liquid at first; thicken it as the pups develop.

WEANING

When puppies approach weaning time (5 to 6 weeks), be certain they are eating well; then shut the mother away from her pups for several hours during the day. Finally, allow her to be with them only at night. Reduce her food intake drastically (this way, she won't have enough food to make milk) and on the day of complete weaning, reduce her water supply, too. The whole weaning process should take about a week, aided by the mother's increasing boredom with the whole puppy business—as well as by her negative reaction to those sharp little teeth.

If you follow the above weaning procedure, the bitch will rarely react adversely. However, occasionally the milk supply persists and the breasts become greatly engorged with milk so they feel caked, or hard. If this happens, use our thumb and forefinger to grasp the base of the nipple and squeeze to release milk. Apply hot towels and give a gentle massage several times daily for a day or two to alleviate the congestion. It is a good idea to continue the food restriction at this time, too. If the situation is serious, apply a tight binder to the body to put pressure on the breasts to decrease milk production.

ORPHAN AND DISOWNED PUPS

For physical and social reasons, puppies are best raised by a good mother. However, when this is not possible, they can still be raised successfully.

PRINCIPLES

Provide:
1. Adequate heat.
2. Substitute formula for bitch's milk.
3. Assistance with urine and stool passage.
4. Isolation and rest.

PROCEDURES

1. Provide adequate heat. This is essential, for inadequate heat is the single greatest killer of orphan pups. Without the mother's body heat, puppies should be kept in an incubator, or heated environment of 85° to 90° F. (29° to 32° C.) for the first week; 80° F. (27°C.) the second week, 75° F. (23° C.) the third and fourth weeks, and 70° F. (21° C.) from then on. If available, a thermostatically controlled heat source is best. If not, place a 250-watt infrared heat bulb over the puppy box, so that half of the area is heated. The pups will crawl into or away from the heated area as their needs dictate. Or as an alternative, drape an electric heating pad over the edge of the box so that it hangs down and covers a few inches of the bottom. Do *not* cover the entire floor of the box with the heating pad; puppies may become overheated if they are

in constant contact with the heat source. Radiant heat from above is more effective and safer.

2. The formula to feed orphan pups is much different from cow's milk (see pages 260 and 261). Use a commercially prepared, canned, substitute formula, which you can obtain from a veterinarian or pet store. These products are almost essential to successful feeding. Certainly, they are more convenient. For a reasonable temporary formula for orphan pups use 1 cup of homogenized milk, supplemented with 2 egg yolks. Or use 1 cup of half-and-half.

Almost all of these formulas provide 5 calories per teaspoon. Use one teaspoonful per day for each ounce of puppy. Divide the total daily amount into 3 or 4 feedings. Thus, you would provide a 4-ounce puppy 1 teaspoonful of formula every 6 hours (4 times a day).

Give the formula in a doll's nursing bottle for small breeds or a regular baby bottle for larger ones. To enlarge the hole in the nipple of a baby bottle, insert a heated needle. The milk should drip out slowly when the bottle is inverted. Your veterinarian may give you instructions and special tubing and syringes for giving the formula by stomach tube. *Never feed puppies with an eye dropper!* This can be lethal, as they may inhale the milk into their lungs.

3. Burp the puppy after each feeding, as you would a human infant. Place the pup upright in the palm of your hand and bounce it gently. Massage the stomach gently. Puppies often burp in a comical way!

4. It is necessary to stimulate the puppy after each feeding to help it urinate and pass stool. To stimulate, wash the pup's abdomen, rear legs, and anus with a pledget of cotton moistened with warm water. In a normal situation, the mother would stimulate this reaction by licking the pup with her tongue. After a week this stimulation is no longer necessary as the process becomes automatic.

5. Wash the pups all over with a dampened cloth, to keep them clean and to moisten their skin.

6. If the skin becomes dry, apply a thin film of baby oil to the

coat every few days. The heat of an incubator environment tends to dry the skin.

7. Watch the puppies' sleeping habits. Like all babies, healthy puppies spend a lot of time sleeping during the first few weeks of their lives. If they do not, it is a sign of trouble. They should eat and sleep.

8. If possible, keep the orphan puppies separated in tiny pens within the whelping box, for the first 10 days. The separation is not essential, but it is desirable. Since the pups do not nurse, they need to satisfy their sucking reflexes and so will suckle one another's tails, feet, and ears, often producing severe irritations.

9. Keep the puppies isolated. It is important that they be left alone and kept away from other animals and from people who might handle them. This is important to prevent possible transmission of disease. Children, especially, can unintentionally be almost brutal in the way they handle young pups. You do neither a pup nor a child a favor by letting them get together at too early an age!

Reproductive Problems of Cats

Most of the troublesome conditions discussed under reproductive problems of dogs also affect cats. They are often managed in the same way—so read the preceding section carefully. Special differences pertaining to cats are described here.

BREEDING

Many people who own a cat know little about their pet's reproductive cycle, and some who have thought they owned a male have been surprised to find the cat suddenly mothering a litter of kittens! Breeding doesn't happen only by the light of the moon, but cats, as compared to dogs, do have seasonally variable cycles.

A male cat will reach puberty at about 1 year of age; a female will start her breeding cycle at 5 to 8 months of age, depending on the season of the year. The cycle covers 14 days; the breeding portion lasts 3 to 6 days. In most temperate climates cycling starts in late January and stops in September. However, a few cats cycle all year.

At the beginning of each cycle, the female cat, called a queen, shows signs of being "in heat." She will show a little vulval swelling and mucoid discharge—but no bleeding. However, her social or emotional behavior is often extreme. An unknowing owner may think the cat is sick; she's just lovesick. The queen may be restless, do a lot of "talking" or howling (especially if she is a Siamese) and may show excessive affection for her owner. She will love to be groomed and will arch her back, roll around on the floor, raise her rear quarters, and turn her tail to one side. She may act so "distressed" that the owner is sure she has a stomach ache.

A prolonged courtship and mating rite is often necessary for cats to become fertile, but there is no tie following the breeding. Left to her own devices, a queen will breed several times—and to different males. This is part of the cat's breeding psychology. These rites serve to encourage real battles among the "suitors" and are the cause of many wounds or cat abscesses. The problem is compounded by the fact that cats (especially males) are highly territorial animals by nature and will defend their home areas against strange cats at all costs.

Ovulation occurs only after breeding, and the newly conceived kittens are not attached to the mother's uterus until about 2 weeks later. This is a real time of concern, since illness or any drugs given during this period may affect the pregnancy.

PREGNANCY

Most of the principles described for dog pregnancies apply to cats, as well. The following are comments on some differences.

A cat pregnancy lasts 63 to 65 days (see gestation table, page 259), and kittens born more than a week early rarely survive. Some females will show signs of "heat" while pregnant, although they will not breed. Pregnancy can be diagnosed by palpating (carefully probing with the fingers) the cat's abdomen about 4 weeks after breeding. The pregnant cat's nipples become enlarged and pink; she shows other external signs which are similar to those described for a pregnant bitch.

Signs of labor generally are similar to those of a bitch. Don't check on the queen in labor too often (she is easily disturbed), but if kittens are not produced within 4 hours or if the queen isn't relaxed and "happy," you should seek veterinary advice.

A cat will usually have 3 to 5 kittens in a litter and rarely have trouble queening (giving birth). However, it is absolutely vital to provide a secluded place for the expectant mother. A cardboard box with high sides, containing a "door" and a cover to maintain darkness is ideal. The box should be supplied with newspapers or cloth scraps for nesting material. It is imperative that you do not disturb the new family for the first 5 to 7 days (no peeking, picking up, patting, or petting). If the kittens are disturbed, some mothers will destroy the entire litter. A nervous queen (especially a Siamese) tends to be more emotional and can become hysterical during or after queening. You may need to provide special sedation and seek advice from your veterinarian on how to handle these cats before they will be able to raise a litter successfully.

THE KITTENS

The general care of kittens is similar to that described for young puppies. Kittens usually nurse at more frequent intervals (every 2 to 3 hours), but like puppies, should gain weight *every* day. Most kittens weigh about 3 ounces at birth and will gain about ⅓ ounce each day—doubling the birth weight by 10 days of age.

If kittens need formula feeding, the commercial milk substitutes made especially for cats are excellent—and the emergency puppy formula (see page 127) works well for kittens, too. Use the same amount of formula per ounce of kitten (one teaspoon) you would for puppies. Feed the kittens with a doll's bottle every 4 hours for the first week. This means that you will divide the total daily amount into 6 portions. Thus a 3-ounce kitten will need ½ to 1 teaspoon of formula at each feeding. It is much more difficult to raise orphan kittens than orphan pups; so pay close attention to details and get veterinary advice if problems develop (see pages 126–128).

Weaning is usually a spontaneous event—well managed by the mother cat. Start feeding the kittens a gruel of milk and kitten food at 4 weeks of age. It should be very fluid at first and gradually thickened with dry cat food as the kittens develop. By 7 weeks they are usually weaned. In a few cases the mother may allow the kittens to continue nursing for many months. The only way you can terminate this practice is to isolate the mother cat for 10 to 14 days, on short rations, so her supply of milk ceases.

21.

Birds and Exotic Pets

Cage Birds

To enjoy good health, birds require good-quality food, regularly cleaned premises, and constantly controlled environmental temperature, light, humidity, and ventilation. They must also have protection from marauding cats and dogs and even from people who would handle them excessively. Escape-proof cages prevent such accidents as cuts and broken bones, but some birds that enjoy flight cages maintain better health by the increased exercise.

ILLNESS IN BIRDS

At any sign of illness, the first thing to do is check all the points of routine care to see if there have been any changes—spoiled food and cold drafts, for example. Resist the temptation to try "cure-all" mixtures for treating loss of appetite, feathers, or voice.

Although birds are often hardy creatures, cold, dampness, drafts, cramped quarters, and—especially—inadequate quantities of food lower their resistance and may precipitate illness.

SIGNS AND SYMPTOMS OF ILLNESS

1. General inactivity or sleepiness.
2. Decreased appetite.
3. Decreased singing, talking, or chirping.
4. Partially closed eyes.
5. Diarrhea or abnormal color or consistency of droppings.

6. Ruffled feathers (indicative of chilling—the most outstanding symptom of illness).

Any of the above symptoms should be considered serious. Get prompt diagnosis and treatment. Until this is available, follow the guidelines below.

FIRST AID FOR ILLNESS

1. Remove grit from the floor of the cage.

2. Provide sufficient heat so the bird's feathers lie sleekly against the body—usually 80° to 90° F. (27° to 32° C.). To do this, suspend the cage several inches above a heating pad or radiator. Drape 75 to 90 percent of the cage with a towel or cover to retain heat. Place an indoor thermometer in the cage and adjust the towel cover (open or close it) until the thermometer registers the desired temperature. *Never* place a bird in direct sunlight, as this may overheat and kill the patient.

3. Help the bird to rest by darkening the room. If the cage has a towel cover and the bird is in a quiet, dark environment, it will usually sleep. About 12 hours of sleep each day is desirable. (Plenty of rest is essential for *all* sick animals.)

4. Improve the diet if possible, as birds must eat constantly to maintain energy. Several days without food can cause death.

5. Keep a daily record of the water the bird is drinking by measuring the total amount of water the water cup holds and comparing this to the amount that remains at the end of the day.

6. Observe and record daily the number and characteristics of the droppings. This information is most helpful if veterinary aid is necessary.

7. Administer *prescribed* medications in the food or in the water. Really sick birds may need to have medication given by stomach tube or injection—but this is a job for your veterinarian.

8. *Do not handle the bird!* The extra stress and struggle produced by inexperienced capture and restraint methods may prove harmful or even fatal to ill birds.

9. Seek veterinary aid early. Sick birds need special care and not all veterinarians have the necessary skills and equipment. It pays to locate your bird's veterinarian *before* you need him.

FIRST AID FOR INJURY

1. Fractures and wounds in birds usually occur from fright, accidental rough handling, or accidents during an escape. Cradle an injured bird in your hands and place it in a small, cotton- or cloth-lined box for transportation to the veterinarian. Try to prevent all attempts at flying or excessive movement by placing the bird in the dark.

2. Do not handle the bird any more than is absolutely necessary.

3. Blood losses of more than a few drops may be serious in small birds, such as budgies and canaries. Gently press a gauze pad or facial tissue onto the bleeding surface to help stop the loss of blood.

4. Birds are very fragile and injuries can easily be aggravated. Leave treatment to the veterinarian.

CAPTURE OF AN ESCAPED BIRD

1. Close all household doors and windows immediately.

2. Leave the bird's cage door open. The bird may return to the cage voluntarily, since that is "home."

3. Darken the room. The bird will become confused and quiet and can usually be picked up easily.

4. In a house, try to "herd" the bird back to the area near the cage. If the bird is kept moving, it will become tired and want to

rest. Within a brief time you will be able to pick the bird up and place it back in the cage.

5. As an alternative, drop a lightweight cloth or net over the bird. Capture by this method is easy and safe.

FEATHER PROBLEMS

Feathers are high-protein protective structures, and they usually reflect the bird's general health. They should be sleek (not ruffled) and bright in color. Feather problems result from a great number of causes.

Molting (loss of feathers) normally takes place periodically in nature, but the artificial atmosphere of a home, with its controlled temperature and light, upsets the natural rhythms and may drastically change molting patterns. Caged birds often receive only marginal nutrition, and they rarely mate. All these factors influence a bird's plumage.

Feather picking, pulling, or chewing may be caused by psychological factors, parasites, nutritional deficiencies, or endocrine abnormalities. Oil on the feathers causes them to mat and lose their insulating value. Oil-soaked birds, therefore, rapidly become chilled and may die.

MANAGEMENT OF FEATHER PROBLEMS

1. Protect birds from excessive exposure to artificial light. Let them go to sleep at night when the sun goes down.

2. Improve nutrition by giving multivitamins in the drinking water daily; providing cuttlebone, oyster shells, or salt blocks; and by feeding a variety of foods. Depending on the species of your bird, you might include raisins, peanut butter, and eggs, as well as several types of seeds, fruits, vegetables, cereals, and even meats.

3. Reduce potentially harmful psychological factors by providing a large cage (to allow physical activity); bells, toys, novelties, or even a companion bird if necessary. The noise from radio or television may also help (seriously)! Relocation of the cage in the

home also may have considerable effect on a lonely, depressed bird.

4. Control feather picking by placing a paper tube or collar around the bird's neck for several months.

5. See your veterinarian for proper treatment and medication for lice, fleas, and mites. These appear as tiny white, gray, or red specks on the feathers, cage, or perches.

6. Treat oil-soaked birds as described below.

Oil-Soaked Birds

These birds, usually wild species, will be chilled, starved, in shock, and often suffering from the toxic effect of the oil. Even a small spot of oil on the breast feathers reduces their insulation value and will produce severe heat loss.

FIRST AID FOR OIL-SOAKED BIRDS

1. Conserve the bird's body heat. This is vital. Place the bird in a small cardboard box with a soft, warm cloth or bedding on the bottom. Provide additional heat if any source is available. You can place a plastic or glass bottle of hot water in the box as an additional heat source.

2. Promptly transport the bird to an appropriate public-health facility (if it is a wild bird) or veterinary hospital, since sophisticated treatment will be necessary to save the patient. Special injections and medications are needed to correct the shock and malnutrition that are usually present.

3. Never use organic liquid solvents (alcohol, ether, etc.). These do a thorough job of removing oil, but they are dangerous. Use diluted liquid household detergents in an emergency. After cleansing the bird, rinse it with plain water and dry it with a stream of warm air (use a blow dryer). It may take several weeks

for complete recovery, since complications from the cleaning are likely. With proper veterinary care, about 50 percent of oil-soaked birds can be expected to recover.

Wild Birds

Almost all wild birds are protected by federal laws, so that they cannot be kept as pets without the authorization of the Bureau of Sport Fisheries and Wildlife, U.S. Department of the Interior. Local conservation officers (game wardens) can usually give helpful advice on the laws and on the care of many wild creatures. In general, you should leave an orphaned or abandoned animal in its natural environment, wherever you find it. In cases of obvious injury or medical need, observe the following hints on temporary aid.

FIRST AID FOR INJURY

1. Return a young bird to its nest if possible.

2. If this is not possible, keep it in a warm (85° F./29° C.), dark place to allow rest and quiet.

3. Feed a weak bird with an eyedropper. Use ¼ to 1 teaspoonful of the following mixture *every hour*: 1 teaspoon of sugar dissolved in 5 teaspoons of water or fortified skim milk. This is also a good diet for hummingbirds.

4. If you must force-feed a bird, use a thin strip of cardboard or a round-ended chopstick to place a semi-soft mash of food in the bird's mouth every hour. Use a dropper to give the bird water every hour. As a bird gains strength, it will usually begin to eat voluntarily—a hopeful sign. Caring for wild birds for more than a few days requires special food and special expertise, but the following foods are good in an emergency.

Basic foods for wild birds are either meats or grains. The meats you can use include strained beef baby food, boiled chicken, hard-boiled eggs, canned dog food, and live insects (such as mealworms). The grains can include dry baby cereal, powdered cornflakes, oatmeal, and wheat germ meal. Other foods include shelled sunflower seeds, peanuts, noncitrus fruits, and berries.

Feed fruit-eaters soaked currants, raisins, or other noncitrus fruits or berries. Birds of prey recover best when fed freshly killed chicks or mice. Large water birds can be fed whole fish, while small water birds can be fed any of the meat foods named above mixed with raw egg yolk. Water birds should have access to or be placed in water for proper eating and bowel elimination. For seed-eaters, mix the meat foods and the grain foods together, with 1 part meat to 5 parts grain. For insect-eaters, the proportion is 1 part meat to 2 parts grain. Add small amounts of ripe banana to the above mixtures to improve the texture and food value.

CLASSIFICATION OF WILD BIRDS (BASED ON EATING HABITS)

Nectar-feeders: hummingbirds
Seed-eaters: sparrows, finches, towhees, and cardinals
Insect-eaters: swallows and flycatchers
Meat-and-fruit-eaters: robins, thrushes, jays, and woodpeckers
Meat-eaters: birds of prey, such as hawks and owls
Fish-eaters: water birds such as gulls, herons, cranes, and grebes
Grain-eaters: water birds such as ducks and geese

The shape of a bird's bill, or beak, is often a guide to the type of food it eats. If you find a bird you cannot identify, consult a bird manual to compare the beaks of the birds classified above to that of your unknown bird. Provide feed accordingly.

If the injured bird begins to eat and has been sick for only a short while, you should release it in an area where similar birds are seen. Your local Audubon Society or conservation officials will be able to advise you on proper procedures.

Wild Amphibians (Salamanders, Frogs, and Toads)

These creatures prefer a cool environment, and in fact, their body temperature is largely dictated by the surrounding environmental temperature. Some amphibians may live for a time in water and as they mature, live both in water and on the land. To provide the necessary moist, cool environment for them, use an enclosure or aquarium that contains a pool of water and a dry area of sand, bark, moss, leaf humus, and forest litter. Never use chlorine in the water, and change it frequently, since uneaten, spoiled food may contaminate it. Do not house amphibians with snakes, snails, or fish, as some species eat others.

Amphibians are usually fed very small amounts several times weekly. Various foods suit various species. Romaine lettuce, ground-up food pellets (the type used for rabbits, guinea pigs, or dogs), minced hard-boiled egg yolk, raw beef, or liver make acceptable foods. If you plan to keep an amphibian for a long period of time, you will need more specific details on care (see suggested reading list in the Appendix).

Wild Reptiles

Turtles, crocodilians, lizards, and snakes are reptiles that are sometimes kept as pets. Some are large or poisonous and thus may be dangerous to humans. It is not wise to keep wild reptiles as pets. However, I will give a few general hints for temporary housing and nursing care that may rehabilitate ill wild reptiles. When they recover, you should release them in their natural habitat.

TURTLES

Turtles are classified as marine, freshwater (semi-aquatic), or land turtles. Marine turtles are seldom seen, but freshwater and land turtles (tortoises) may be found and housed quite satisfactorily for a short time. They thrive in warmth (75° to 80° F./23°

to 29° C.) and require an environment no cooler than 71° F. (21° C.).

Turtles may be kept in a terrarium or a box containing rocks or gravel for a dry-land area and a recessed pan of water for a pool. Use an overhead light to provide heat. Some sunlight during the day is beneficial.

Turtles need a variety of foods and will usually eat lettuce, apples, earthworms, insects, fish, chopped lean meat, cheese, or canned dog food. Ant eggs, commonly sold for turtle food, are an inadequate diet. Put food for small turtles in their water every other day (twice a week as they grow larger). Change the water frequently to keep it clean.

To treat turtles with soft shells, add cod-liver oil, ground egg-shells, or ground fish to the diet. To treat turtles with sore eyes, add cod-liver oil to the food, provide additional sunlight, or apply swabs of boric acid solution or warm tea to the eyes once a day.

CROCODILIANS

Small alligators and crocodiles, which inhabit the southern United States, and South American caimans are often sold as pets. To handle these reptiles, grasp them behind the head and by the base of the tail. They will thrive in the terrarium environment described for turtles but do better at warmer temperatures of 80° to 90° F. (27° to 32° C.). They will eat raw, lean meat, fish, or minnows and should be fed twice weekly. Put the food in their water.

LIZARDS

Lizards are found throughout the world. Their needs vary from species to species, but most need warmth 85° to 90° F. (29° to 32° C.) and good sunlight. Many lizards eat insects (flies, grubs), mealworms, or earthworms, but some eat fruit, buds, and berries. All these reptiles should be fed daily—usually at noon, when light and temperature intensities are high. Most lizards have low water requirements; a small amount of water sprinkled on the rocks in the pen each day is sufficient for some, while a tiny pool is desirable for others.

SNAKES

Snakes inhabit all types of terrain. They can be gentle and tame—especially if you handle them frequently. To do so, grasp them behind the head with one hand and support their bodies with the other. Always make slow, deliberate movements so as not to excite or frighten them. You can easily transport them in a cloth sack, such as a pillow case. Snakes do best at temperatures of 75° to 85° F. (23° to 29° C.). They should be housed in escape-proof, wire-screen-covered boxes or glass tanks. The housing should be *dry;* provide a sand floor, with some tree bark to hide under, and a small pan of water. All snakes are meat-eaters. A weekly feeding of earthworms, insects, and lean beef is adequate for small snakes. Large snakes only feed several times a year. They swallow whole prey, such as chicks, mice, and frogs. Cannibalism is a common trait for some species so they are usually best housed alone. For further information on reptiles, alligators, and lizards, consult the reading list in Appendix 9 (page 265).

II.

FIRST AID TECHNIQUES

22.

The First Aid Kit

The drugs and equipment needed for each species varies. The list here is appropriate for dogs or cats, but it includes only the essentials. It is assumed that common household items such as scissors, pliers, blankets, soap, baking soda, and mineral oil are readily available.

The contents of this first aid kit (see Figure 10, page 144) should provide material to help restrain a hysterical patient and to treat major problems such as bleeding, wounds, shock, heatstroke, poisoning, and eye injuries. The parenthetical numbers in the following list indicate the quantity.

Contents for a Pet First Aid Kit

Materials and Equipment
Gauze bandages, 1″ and 2″ rolls (1 each)
Gauze dressing pads, 3″ × 3″ (8)
Adhesive tape, 1″ roll (1)
Cotton batting roll (1)
Triangular bandage (1)
Rectal thermometer (1)
Q-tips (6)
Tweezers (1)

Medications
3% hydrogen peroxide (2 oz.)
Milk of magnesia tablets, 5 gr. (10)
Activated charcoal tablets (20)
Kaolin mixture (2 oz.)
Antibacterial ointment
    For eye—⅛-oz. tube (1)
    For skin—⅛-oz. tube (1)

Be sure to keep replacing the materials and medications as you use them.

FIGURE 10. *A pet first aid kit.*

Top row: Empty plastic storage box.

Second row: Muslin bandage, sterile 3″ x 3″ gauze compresses, 3 1-ounce bottles of Kaolin-pectin diarrhea medication, 2 packages of iodine wound-dressing medication, 1 ⅛-ounce tube of ophthalmic ointment.

Third row: Roll of cotton, 2″ and 1″ gauze bandages, small sterile 2″ x 2″ gauze compresses, 2-ounce bottle of 3% hydrogen peroxide, package of activated charcoal tablets, jar of topical antibiotic ointment.

Fourth row: Nonsterile gauze compresses, small tweezers, nonstick plastic wound strips, scissors, package of Milk of Magnesia tablets, 1″ roll of adhesive tape, Q-tips, rectal thermometer in plastic case.

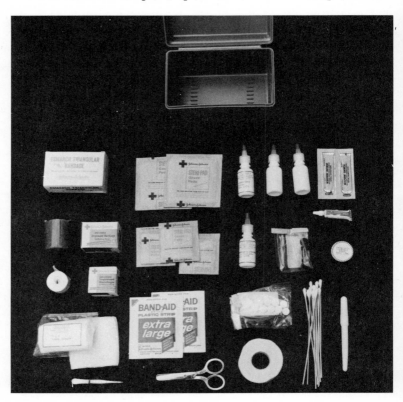

23.

Rescue and Transport
of Injured Animals

Rescue is a procedure for moving an animal from a dangerous location to a place of safety.

Like people, pets can get themselves into many dangerous predicaments. They may fall through ice, swim in dangerous rivers, jump into swimming pools they cannot get out of, get trapped in narrow pipes or between buildings, fall off cliffs or fire escapes, and even climb trees and then be afraid to descend. They can also become trapped in abandoned wells, blazing buildings, and discarded boxes or refrigerators.

Principles for animal rescue are similar to those used to save people. Success in great measure depends on the rescuer's having a cool head, common sense, ingenuity, and bravery.

I worked closely with officers of a humane organization in a large metropolitan city for several years. It was truly amazing how these experienced men were able to use catch-sticks, coaxing, and coercion to rescue trapped and injured pets.

Principles of Rescue

1. Let professionals do it (if they are available).

2. Do not risk human life or limb on behalf of animals—especially wild species.

3. Take time to plan the rescue and to appeal for professional assistance. This applies in all cases *except* in dire emergencies (fire, drowning, asphyxia, or profuse bleeding).

4. In the case of dire emergency (see above), administer the

appropriate first aid on the spot. Then move the patient to a location a short distance away from danger, where you can apply more expert care. Finally, transport the patient to a veterinary hospital for more definitive treatment.

    5. *Use the following emergency first aid measures:*
      a. Clear airway.
      b. Give artificial respiration.
      c. Control bleeding.
      d. Check for other injuries.
      e. Immobilize injured limbs.
      f. Transport to safety.

Procedures for Safe Transport

    1. Methods of transport used depend on the size, temperament, and injuries of the patient, the help available, the distance to be traveled, and whether or not the animal is conscious.

    2. Muzzle the patient if it is conscious and capable of biting.

    3. If the patient must be pulled or dragged, carefully grasp the skin at the top of the neck near the head, and at the shoulders, and pull the animal, head first. Keep the body in a straight line and keep it moving. Be sure the legs hang naturally and slide along freely. If possible, gently slide the patient onto a board or blanket; this will ease the move and prevent further injury. Do not bend or twist the animal, especially if there is any evidence of injury to the spine or limbs.

    4. Support any obviously injured or deformed part by holding it carefully, with your hands placed above *and* below the injured area. Try to immobilize injured limbs with temporary splints (see pages 110–111). The first aid adage, "splint them where they lie," is appropriate for animals, as well as for humans.

    5. Keep an injured animal in a reclining position at all times if possible. If it is unconscious, this may be easy; you will have no trouble strapping it to a board or other improvised stretcher or lifting it in a blanket, then placing it in a warm vehicle for transportation to a veterinary hospital.

6. Transport a less seriously injured animal in a shipping crate, cat basket or carrier, or even a large box.

7. Be calm, reassuring, and firm; keep the patient quiet, lying down, and warm.

Special Rescue Problems

1. An animal trapped in a well, pit, or on a cliff can often be rescued with a lasso. The rope loop works especially well for a smaller animal (under 60 pounds; 27 kilograms). If you can get the loop around the animal's neck and gently tighten until it cannot slip over the head, rescue is usually assured. Tighten the rope gently until it is taut. Call to the animal, and as it scrambles to climb up the steep wall, pull firmly and rapidly on the rope. You will not asphyxiate or "hang" the pet. Its neck is strong, and your action will be brief but helpful. This method is surprisingly successful—once you get the noose on the neck.

A noose on the end of a long pole (10 to 12 feet) is a most versatile implement to have on hand. With it you can get an animal down from a tree (especially if you also have a ladder), pull one from ice or out of a pool, and handle many other baffling rescue problems.

2. A cat in a tree will usually come down with some coaxing, especially if you entice it with a dish of strong-smelling fish when it becomes hungry.

3. Do not approach or in any way aggravate a skunk that temporarily invades a garage, basement, or other building. Leave the doors open and place canned dog food, raw eggs, or other similar food outside. When night falls, the skunk will leave quietly.

4. Spray liquid soap or soapy water on a pet that is stuck in a narrow pipe or building space. This may lubricate the animal enough so that you can pull it out or it can wiggle free. Remember, a cat uses its whiskers to judge the width of a narrow opening. If the whiskers fit through, the cat's body can, too—so *never* trim your cat's whiskers. Your pet could misjudge the size of an opening.

5. Electrical emergencies usually occur when an animal bites through an appliance or lamp cord. Pull the cord out of the wall or turn off the switch controlling that circuit. If your pet has contacted a downed live wire, use a *long, dry* pole or a *dry* rope to pull the animal from the wire or the wire from the animal. This can be dangerous, so be sure that your hands are dry and that you are standing on something dry. Even low voltages in a home can be very dangerous—so use extreme care. Patients that have been exposed to electric currents usually need prompt artificial respiration (see pages 14–16) and immediate veterinary care.

6. Do not enter a burning or gas-filled building to try to rescue your pet—it is just too dangerous. Professional fire, emergency, and utility officials will soon be on the scene. Await their services!

24.

Restraint

Anyone who reads this book loves animals or at least is vitally interested in their welfare. In most instances the first-aider will be faced with a patient that does not recognize such love and concern. Injured animals hurt. They are afraid and do not understand what has happened to make them hurt. Thus, their master or friend, who may have unintentionally caused the injury, no longer seems trustworthy and their natural instincts tell them to escape and hide. Failing this, they tend to strike out at anyone who approaches, for they fear their painful experience will be repeated.

If the first-aider understands this instinctive behavior and knows how to deal with it psychologically, as well as physically, he can usually help prevent further pain and avoid personal injury.

In veterinary medicine, tranquilizers, sedatives, and anesthetics make care of injured animals easier and more humane than it was just a few years ago. However, one must get the patient to the veterinary hospital for proper selection and administration of one of these medications. In the time between the injury and arrival at the hospital, the first-aider must use his best efforts to alleviate the animal's suffering.

Principles of Restraint

1. Approach the patient with a firm but kind and quiet manner. Use its name if you know it and allow the animal to sniff the back of your closed fist.

2. Do nothing to further injure the patient.

3. Restrain the patient in a way that will not allow it to injure *itself*.

4. Protect *yourself* from injury that may be inflicted upon you by the patient.

5. Place the animal in a situation different from its usual secure environment (e.g., on the top of a table instead of on the floor). The newness will create uncertainty but not pain, and the patient will be more cooperative and thus easier to treat.

Procedures for Dogs

MUZZLING A DOG

Many dogs do not need muzzling, but if you must handle a strange or injured dog or if you have any doubt about its disposition, always apply a muzzle. This is not uncomfortable for the dog, and it ensures safety for the first-aider. In addition, muzzled dogs seem to realize they have been rendered harmless, and they often accept handling that they might otherwise reject.

1. Use a length of heavy cord, bandage, or cloth tape. Loop it around the jaws, just behind the dog's nose, and tie it with a half hitch under the chin. (See Figure 11.) Make several additional turns around the jaws. Bring the ends back behind the ears and tie them in a firm bow knot. (See Figure 12.) It may be necessary to have an assistant hold the dog's head and neck while you apply the muzzle. He may also have to hold the patient's front legs so the animal cannot scratch the muzzle off before you can tie it securely. Wire or leather basket muzzles are seldom satisfactory for this purpose.

2. Dogs with short necks and faces need special muzzling. Fold a thick towel lengthwise and wrap it around the animal's neck. Hold the ends firmly behind the dog's head and ears. This simple, comfortable collar will keep the head facing forward, effectively restraining the dog so that it cannot turn and bite you (see Figure 21, page 158).

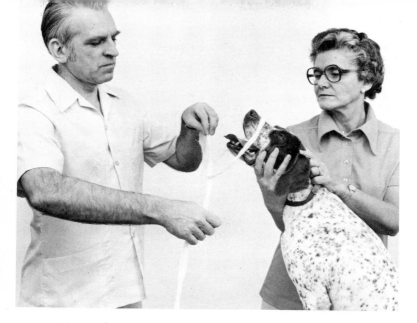

FIGURE 11. *Applying a muzzle.* Use a length of heavy cord, bandage, or cloth tape. Loop it around the patient's nose and mouth.

FIGURE 12. *Completing the muzzle.* Wrap the bandage around the dog's muzzle several times and tie the ends behind the ears using a bow knot.

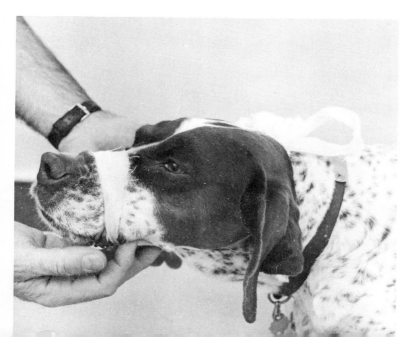

PICKING UP A DOG AND
PLACING IT ON A TABLE

1. Approach the dog in a friendly and cautious manner.
2. Make sure its collar is snug.
3. Position the dog between you and the table.
4. Stand on the dog's left side, facing the table.
5. Grasp the leash with your left hand and pull the dog gently toward the table.
6. Place your right arm all the way over the dog's back and grasp the chest on the far side. Support the breastbone with your right hand. Lift with both arms and swing the dog up and onto the table with one smooth motion. (See Figure 13.)
7. If you are lifting a very large dog, have a second person lift the hind quarters simultaneously.
8. Caress the dog and speak quietly to it, so that it feels reassured about being on the table.
9. To lift a very small or uncooperative dog, fold a heavy blanket several times and drop it over the patient. You can then pick the dog up by the shoulders and place it on the table. (This method also works well for cats.) The patient feels secure hidden in the blanket, and the blanket will serve as padding to protect the handler.

CARRYING A DOG

1. To pick up a small dog, grasp the collar with your left hand, and place your right arm all the way over the back and around under the chest on the far side (see Figure 14). This arm serves to cradle the dog's body against your chest. Try to grasp one or both of the front legs in your right hand, as this will make the dog feel secure and comfortable. If it feels secure in your arms, it tends to relax. (See Figure 15.)
2. Pick up a larger dog in the same manner (see figures 16–19, pages 156–157), except cross your left arm under the dog's neck and grasp its right shoulder or elbow. Press the dog's shoulder

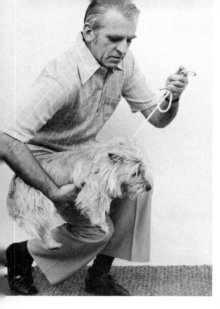 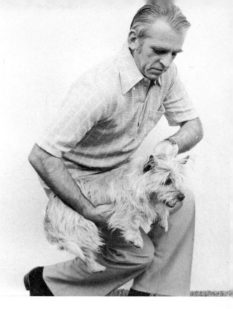

FIGURE 13 (left). *Lifting a small dog.* Hold the leash firmly to keep the dog's head extended. Place your dominant hand under its chest and lift smoothly and quickly. The same maneuver may be accomplished by holding the dog's collar firmly (see FIGURE 14, right). In either case, coordinate both hands to hold the dog firmly and safely.

FIGURE 15. *Carrying a small dog.* As you lift the dog from the floor, tuck it under your arm, and press it securely against your body. Held firmly, it will feel safe and relax. Hold the dog's elbow nearest your body firmly for additional stability.

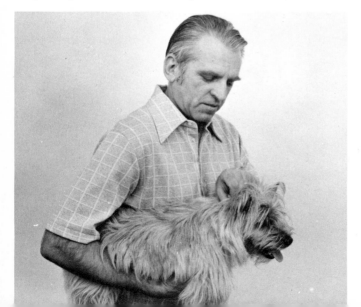

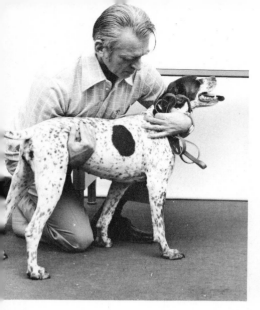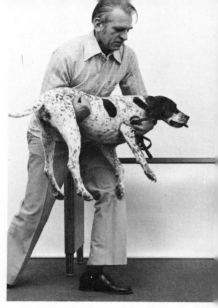

FIGURE 16 (left). *Lifting a large dog.* Crouch beside the dog. Place one arm around the neck and the other arm under the abdomen.
FIGURE 17 (right). Lift smoothly and swing the dog up to a table.

FIGURE 18. *Alternate method for lifting and holding a large dog.* Place one arm around the dog's neck, grasping its elbow with your hand. Place the other arm around the dog's hindquarters and grasp the rear leg. Snuggle the dog close to your body.

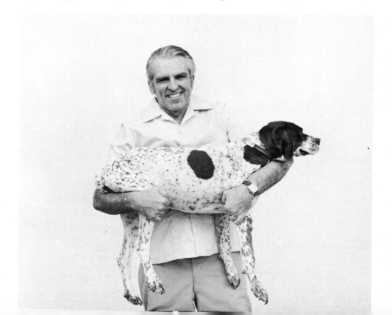

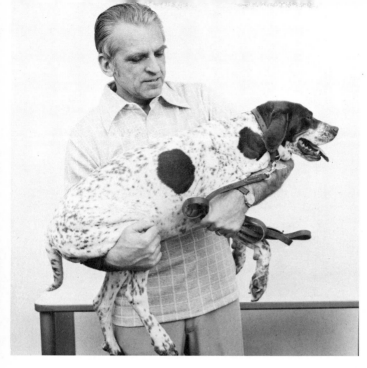

FIGURE 19. Hold the hindquarters lower, so that the dog "sits" on your arm.

against your chest. With your right arm, cradle the dog under its rump (tail) to hold the legs together and press the dog's entire body against your chest. This will be easier if you grasp the dog's right hind leg with your right hand. Lift smoothly, keeping the rear legs lower so that the dog is almost sitting on its buttocks on your forearm. As an alternative, for a female dog, place your right arm under the dog's abdomen.

HOLDING A DOG FOR EXAMINATION OR TREATMENT

1. Wrap a small dog in a blanket with only its head exposed. As an alternative, restrain the head by grasping the collar and neck just behind the head. In either case, "hug" the animal's body

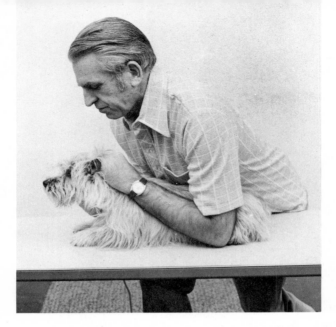

FIGURE 20. *Holding a dog for examination or administration of oral medication.* Place the dog on a table. Hold its collar and neck and "hug" the animal against your chest, keeping it gently confined between your arms, your body, and the table.

FIGURE 21. *Holding a more active patient.* Use a heavy towel or blanket to further restrict the patient's head.

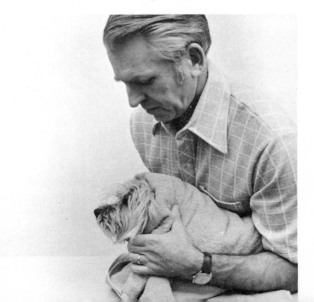

against your chest for further support and confinement. (See figures 20 and 21.)

2. In some cases it may be desirable to restrain the dog on its side—e.g., when bandaging its feet or legs or cutting its toenails. To position, reach over the top of the patient's back and grasp the legs nearest your body from the table, press it against your chest and gently roll it down onto the table top. Use your hands to hold the legs down, your arm to press the dog's neck gently to the table, and your chest to help keep the dog's body down. The patient will be confined comfortably and securely, but its legs will be free for examination and treatment. (See figures 22 and 23, page 160.)

3. Particularly aggressive or vicious dogs should be handled only by professional humane-society officers, police, or veterinary personnel. If you are obliged to face such an animal, these hints may be useful:

    a. Few dogs will actually attack, but if one does, use an ordinary straight chair to block the animal and keep it away so you will not be bitten.

    b. Place two leashes (or lassos) around the animal's neck and have two people on opposite sides hold them. This may prevent the animal from moving toward either holder. Have a third person attempt to apply a muzzle or place a blanket over the dog's neck and shoulders for safe and humane confinement of its head.

    c. Use a padded dog stick. This is a pole with a slip-noose attached to the end. Place the noose around the animal's neck and secure it. This will enable you to hold the dog away and lead it to a confining cage, animal ambulance, or other place for treatment. These "catchers" also are helpful in holding a dog to apply a muzzle. (See figures 24 and 25, page 161.)

Procedures for Cats

In general, the cat is a very independent creature. It has a personality that differs markedly from a typical dog's. For this reason,

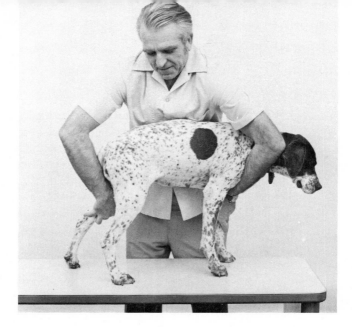

FIGURE 22. *Restraining a dog on its side*. Place the dog on its side on a table by reaching over the dog as shown. Pull its legs away and slide it down your body to the table. Two people working together can accomplish this more easily.

FIGURE 23. *Confining the dog on the table*. Hold the legs extended and press the neck gently to the table with your arm.

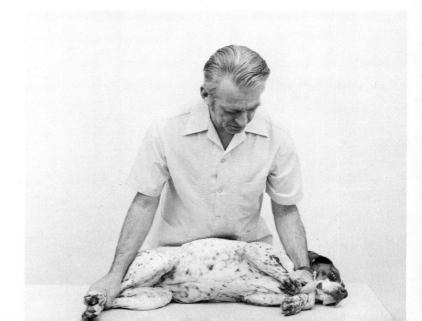

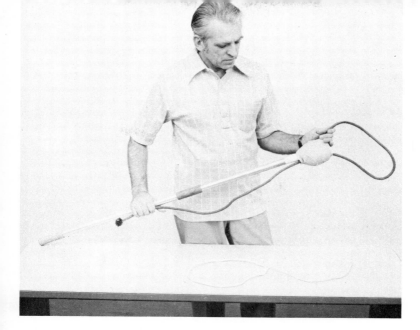

FIGURE 24. *Restraint ropes*. Use the rope lasso shown on the table as a leash.

FIGURE 25. *The padded stick*. Use the padded stick to keep a vicious patient at a distance. This tool is used by humane-society officers for safely handling a strange or aggressive animal.

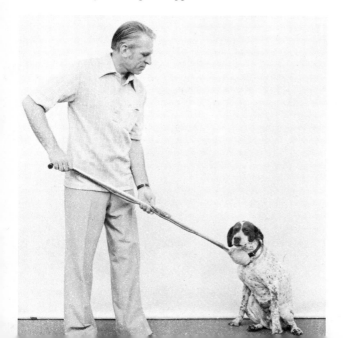

cats must either be restrained very securely and almost forcibly or confined to an area where they think they are free but in reality are not. The cat also has five points that may cause the first-aider harm: the mouth, which may bite, and the four feet, which can cause painful scratches. It is almost impossible to muzzle a cat, so restraint of the feet is the paramount goal.

To humanely "disarm" the cat's claws, secure the two front legs together, just above the feet, by winding adhesive tape around them two or three times. Then fasten the rear legs together in a similar manner. Hold the head firmly. The cat can now be examined and treated carefully and effectively. (See Figure 26.)

Actually, the cat is usually a bluffer and it will respond well to confident but firm handling. It is also forgetful and forgiving. If a

FIGURE 26. *Using adhesive tape to control a cat.* Fasten the two front legs, then the two rear legs, together. This safely and effectively disarms a cat, making examination or treatment easier.

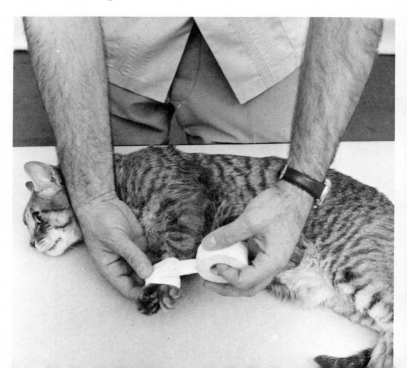

cat becomes angry at forced treatment, release it. Within a few minutes it will once again be docile and approachable.

PICKING UP OR CARRYING A CAT

1. Reassure the cat. Talk to it quietly, gently stroke its head and ears, and run your hand down its back.

2. Place one hand over the cat's back and pick it up by grasping it under the chest (sternum). With your other hand, either grasp the scruff of the neck or cradle the cat under the neck. Rest the cat's lower body on your forearm and snuggle the cat against your body. (See Figure 27).

3. Transport a cat in a cat basket or carrier, or cloth bag, such as a pillow case or canvas or burlap bag, tied closed. The cat

FIGURE 27. *Picking up and carrying a cat.* Place one hand under the chest and grasp the front legs. Cradle the neck in the other hand and rest the cat on your forearm, holding it firmly but not forcibly.

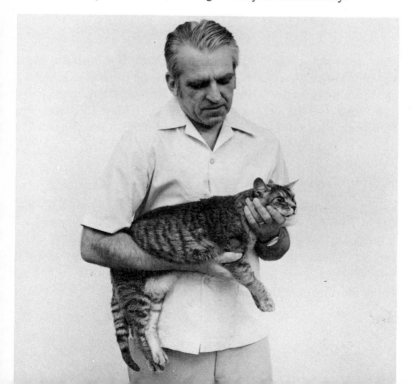

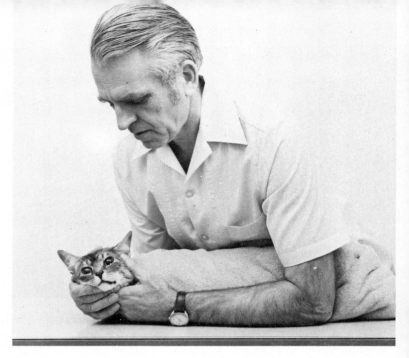

FIGURE 28. *Restraining an unruly, or vicious cat.* Wrap the cat in a heavy towel or blanket.

cannot see out and will feel snug and secure. If the head is to be examined or oral medication given, loosen the bag and expose only the head; this effectively restrains the patient in the bag.

4. Many of the general restraint methods described for dogs will work with the usual docile cat. Try them. (See pages 154–159.)

RESTRAINING UNRULY OR VICIOUS CATS

1. In most instances, an unruly or vicious cat can be controlled with a folded blanket or thick towel. Drop the blanket over the cat in its box or cage and pick up the animal inside the blanket. With the cat rolled in the blanket and only a foot or the head protruding, you can apply medication or bandages without danger to either the patient or the handler. (See Figure 28.)

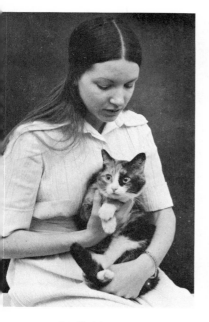 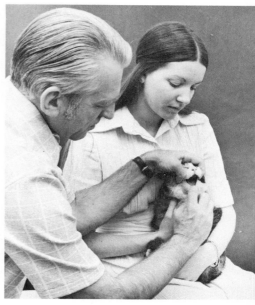

FIGURE 29 (left). *Restraining a quiet cat.* Hold the cat on your lap, restraining all four legs as demonstrated.

FIGURE 30 (right). *Restraining a cat for examination or administration of medication.*

2. Use thick leather or canvas work gloves when handling a truly aggressive cat. Remember, cats will scratch and bite severely, and they will almost always attack your face or hands. Place these obstreperous patients in a strong bag or cat box and take them to the veterinary hospital, where drugs can be used for restraint. This is safer, wiser, and more humane.

EXAMINATION OF DOCILE CATS

To examine a quiet cat, place the cat in your lap and hold it firmly (see figures 29 and 30).

25.

Dressings and Bandages

Applying a dressing and bandage to an animal with a hairy coat is very different from applying these to human skin. In particular, adhesive gauze and Band-Aids do not stick to hair, so these should not be used. Ideally, before any wound is dressed, you should clip the affected area of skin free of hair and cleanse it. Then cover the area with a sterile gauze dressing. Further protect this dressing with a thin layer of cotton or other padding. Then bandage the entire area to hold the material firmly in place.

When sterile dressing materials are not available, you must use improvised substitutes. Strips of cotton sheeting, muslin, handkerchiefs, towels, plastic-bag material, or even paper towels will serve in an emergency. The object is to protect the wound from further contamination until you can apply proper dressings. *Never* use cotton batting directly on an open wound, since the lint will adhere to the tissues and make later wound-cleaning difficult. However, once the wound is covered, cotton may be used.

In most first aid situations, it is not possible to clip the hair away from the open wound. If this is the case, use a damp cloth to wet and wipe the hair away. Gently remove any gross debris. Then cover the wound with sterile gauze or a clean cloth. Reinforce this with a padding of cotton, toweling, or strips of thin blanket material. Finally, bandage the dressing and tape or pin it firmly. You may use strips of cloth for the bandage, but these substitutes are not nearly as good as rolls of gauze bandage and/or adhesive tape for completing the protective wound cover. The adhesive tape will adhere to the bandaging and will usually hold it firmly in place.

Dressings

DEFINITION

Dressings are the material in direct contact with the wound. Sterile gauze pads or plastic-film-covered pads are most desirable, but a clean, nonsterile cloth, handkerchief, or towel will be adequate. To sterilize a nonsterile cloth, wrap it in aluminum foil and bake in a 350-degree oven for three hours. This is acceptable if you are changing dressings daily and sterile materials are not available to you. However, it is better to buy commercially prepared, packaged sterile dressings for your first aid kit.

FUNCTIONS

1. To protect the wound and control bleeding.
2. To absorb blood and wound secretions.
3. To prevent contamination.
4. To reduce pain.

Bandages

DEFINITION

Bandages usually are strips of cloth material used to hold dressings or splints in place. Larger pieces of cloth may be used as binders to hold dressings in place on a large surface such as the chest or the abdomen. Remember, every wound should be covered *first* with a protective dressing and padding material.

TYPES OF BANDAGES

See Figure 31 (page 168) for illustrations of the following bandages:

1. *Gauze bandages*. These come in 10-yard rolls and are 1, 2, or 3 inches wide. A narrow bandage tends to roll up like a string and may cause local pressure unless it is applied carefully. Gauze bandages are generally used to bandage wounds of the feet, legs, head, and tail.

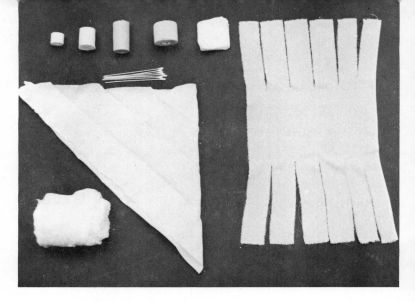

FIGURE 31. *Types of bandages.*
Top: 1″, 2″, and 3″ gauze bandages; 2″ elastic bandage; gauze
  sponges.
Right: Binder (many-tailed muslin bandage).
Left: Q-tips, triangular muslin bandage, roll of cotton padding.

2. *Elastic bandages.* Similar in size and function to the gauze
bandages described above, elastic bandages are recommended
when more pressure is needed. However, they may produce excessive pressure and restrict blood supply unless they are properly
applied.

3. *Triangular muslin bandages.* These bandages, also used in
human first aid kits, can be folded and used for pressure pads.
They may also be used as binders for covering dressings applied to
the head, chest, or abdomen.

4. *Binders* (many-tailed muslin bandages). These are usually
used with abdominal or chest wounds. They are large rectangles of
muslin, with the two opposing short edges torn into narrow pigtail
strips about one-third of the way into each side. The solid portion
is placed over a wound-dressing pad and the free pigtail ends are
brought up and tied over the animal's back.

FUNCTIONS

1. To hold a dressing in place.
2. To support, protect, and immobilize an injured part.

BANDAGING

Bandages must not interfere with circulation. The turns of the bandage should be evenly distributed—firm but not tight. If the bandage is loose, the dressing will slip and be useless.

Bandages must be checked periodically. The patient may chew at or even remove the bandage. Usually, excessive chewing or licking is an indication that the bandage is uncomfortable. Also, the wound may swell so the bandage becomes too tight and obstructs circulation. Or the bandage may shift position and allow the dressing to slip.

The following section on bandaging a foot and an abdomen will demonstrate the techniques you will need for bandaging other body parts, as well.

BANDAGING THE FOOT

The foot bandage (see figures 32–39, pages 170–173) must be firm, adaptable to the flexing of the foot joints, and tough enough to resist the wear of walking. The first-aider will need 1-inch adhesive tape, 2-inch gauze bandage, cotton batting, and gauze dressings.

1. Muzzle and restrain the patient (see pages 151–152 and 157–165) in a comfortable position. Have a helper hold the leg in an extended position.
2. Place a gauze dressing over the cleaned wound; it should extend well beyond the wound on all sides.
3. Pad the spaces between the toes with wisps of cotton to prevent irritation.
4. Wrap the foot with a thin sheet of cotton batting, covering the entire foot and the leg to a point several inches above the foot. Be sure the cotton batting is smooth and free of folds or wadded areas.

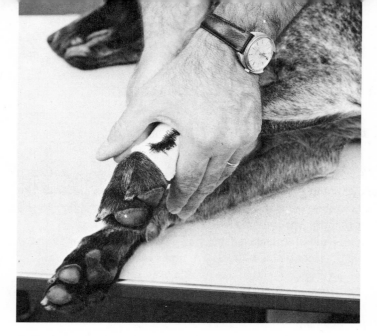

Bandaging a foot.

FIGURE 32. Press sterile gauze dressing over the cleansed wound to help control bleeding.

FIGURE 33. Add cotton for more pressure and padding if needed.

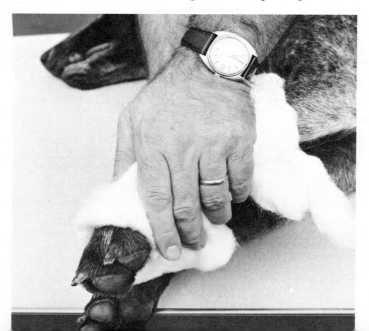

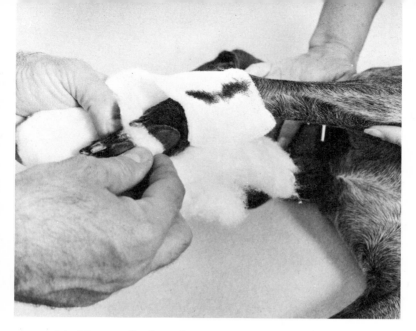

FIGURE 34. Place small wisps of cotton between the toes.

FIGURE 35. Wrap a thin layer of cotton batting around the foot and lower leg. Loop appropriate-width gauze bandage back and forth over the end of the foot.

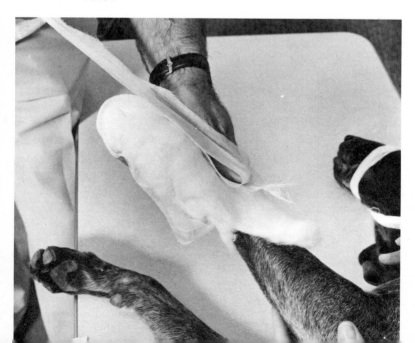

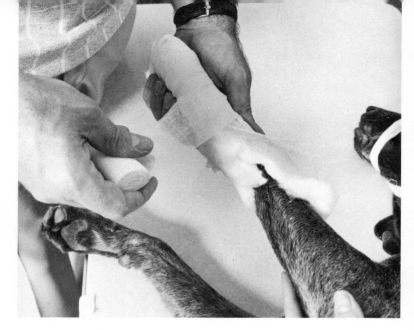

Bandaging a foot.

FIGURE 36. Start at the toes and wrap gauze bandage firmly around the leg in an upward spiral.

FIGURE 37. Tie the gauze at the top of the padded area.

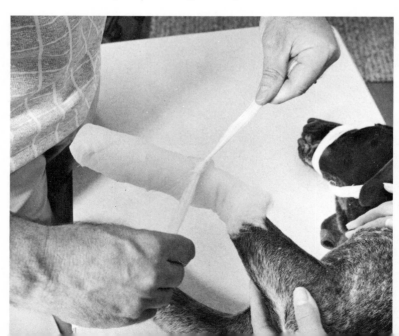

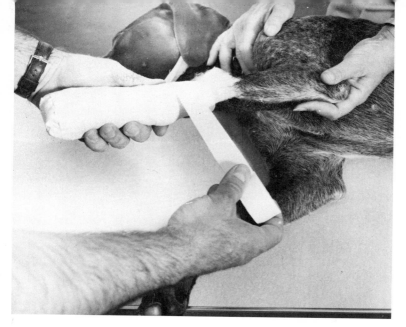

FIGURE 38. Wrap 1″ tape around the leg for additional protection. Apply this in the same manner as the gauze bandage.

FIGURE 39. The finished bandage.

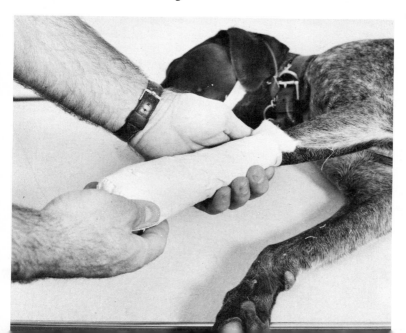

5. Bandage the foot and toes. Using a 2-inch gauze bandage, start near the toes and wrap the bandage back and forth across the bottom of the foot. Next, start at the toes and wind smoothly overlapping rows of bandage around the foot and leg in an upward spiral. Apply the bandage firmly and evenly. To finish the bandage at the top, fold the free end back on itself for 8 to 10 inches, so that the free end comes around one side of the leg while the folded end appears on the other. Then tie the 2 segments together with a square knot.

6. Cover the bandage with 1-inch adhesive tape for additional protection. Cut several 6- to 8-inch strips of tape and use them to "box" the end of the foot. Then wrap adhesive tape around the bandaged leg in a manner similar to that used to apply the bandage. Do not apply it tightly. At the top of the bandage, incorporate a few wisps of adjacent hairs of the leg in the last turn or two of tape. This will help prevent the bandage from slipping down the leg.

BANDAGING THE ABDOMEN

Covering a large wound on the abdomen or chest (see figures 3, 4, pages 24 and 25, and Figure 40) presents a special problem: this area is in constant movement, and the trunk of the body is often tapered so a bandage tends to slip. The basic gauze-bandage procedure used for foot bandages works in this case, as well. However, it requires more material and is difficult to secure properly. The muslin binder will work better for first aid emergencies. The first-aider will need cotton sheeting, muslin or a triangle bandage, cotton padding, and sterile gauze dressings. Adhesive tape may be useful, too.

1. Muzzle and restrain the patient (see pages 151–152 and 159–165) in a comfortable position. If possible, have the animal stand, so that bandages can easily circle the abdomen.

2. Place a gauze dressing over the cleaned wound. It should extend well beyond the wound on all sides. If any internal organs

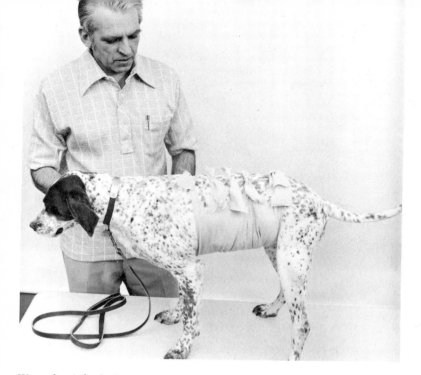

Wounds of the body.

FIGURE 40. Cover cotton with many-tailed muslin bandage and tie the opposing tails over the back. By adjusting each tie, you can apply firm, even pressure to other tapered areas (head, neck, or chest).

are exposed, dampen the dressing material to prevent the tissue from drying out.

3. Place a thin sheet of cotton batting over the dressing and allow it to extend most of the way around the patient's abdomen. (A thin blanket material or a towel can be used as substitute padding.) If more pressure is needed to help control bleeding, place several thicknesses of the padding over the wound area.

4. Prepare a large rectangular piece of muslin or cotton sheeting as a many-tailed bandage to cover the padding and dressing. Make the sheet 12 to 18 inches *wider* than the wounded area and 6 to 8 inches *longer* than the distance around the patient's

abdomen at the widest part. Tear a fringe of 2-inch-wide strips one-third of the way into this latter distance on opposing edges to form tails that you can tie together over the patient's back.

5. Lay the solid center portion of the binder over the padded dressing, pull the tails up snugly, and tie them carefully to produce firm, molded pressure on the entire abdomen. If necessary, apply adhesive tape over the bandage to help add firmness.

Care of Bandaged Wounds

The instructions in this book are for *primary* care; take your pet to a veterinarian as soon as possible for more extensive bandaging and dressing.

Check bandages frequently and change them if they become wet, bloody, or if they slip, or if the patient chews or paws at them excessively. Even if none of these problems is evident, change bandages daily for observation, cleaning, and medication of the wound. Your veterinarian will give you specific advice on these matters, since many wounds require special or extensive dressing.

26.

Administration of Medications

Injections

Special precautions are needed when giving drugs by injection. If this is required, the procedure should be described in detail and demonstrated to you by your veterinarian. Possession of syringes and needles is unlawful except by prescription from a veterinarian.

Oral Medications

GIVING CAPSULES AND TABLETS TO DOGS

You can often hide solid medication in pieces of meat, canned dog food, or cheese. Toss a few unbaited tidbits to the patient; then offer one containing the tablet. The dog will usually accept it. If the dog chews the food, it may be necessary to crush the tablet before hiding it in the tidbit. A discriminating animal will eat the food but spit out the medication. Pets can be clever!

If the patient isn't eating well, you can use the same trick, but you may have to push the tidbit containing the medication down the patient's throat. Still, your pet will usually accept a hidden tablet more readily than it would an undisguised one.

It is generally easy to "pill" a placid dog. Give solid medications quickly and decisively so the pilling is all over before the animal realizes what is happening.

Hold the tablet between the index and middle fingers of your dominant hand. Slip the thumb of your other hand behind the dog's large upper fang tooth and press up on the hard roof of the mouth.

At the same time press down on the lower jaw with the thumb of your dominant hand. Push the pill deeply into the patient's throat. (See Figure 41.) Withdraw your hands quickly, hold the dog's mouth closed, and tap the underside of its chin sharply. The tap usually startles the dog and forces it to swallow the pill. When the dog licks its nose, you can be confident that the medication has been swallowed.

A dog may resist opening its mouth. In this case compress the lips firmly against the teeth. The discomfort causes the patient to open its mouth, and you can then place the tablet inside, as described above. Try to roll the lips inward, over the teeth, as the dog opens its mouth. This obliges the animal to keep its mouth

FIGURE 41. *"Pilling" a dog.* Hold the tablet between the index and middle fingers of your dominant hand. Open the dog's mouth by placing the thumb of your other hand behind the patient's large fang tooth and pressing up on the roof of the mouth. Press down on the dog's lower jaw with the thumb or the two free fingers of the dominant hand. Push the tablet way down the dog's throat. Withdraw your fingers and close the dog's mouth quickly. Tap its nose sharply with your fingers. It will usually swallow the tablet.

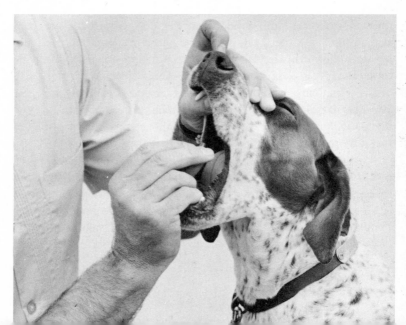

open; otherwise, it will pinch its own lips. The veterinarian may use special pill forceps to give medication to particularly obstreperous patients.

GIVING CAPSULES AND TABLETS TO CATS

Place the cat on a table and hold its head elevated and tipped back. If you are right-handed, use your left hand to hold the head from behind, with the index finger at the corner of the mouth on one side and the thumb at the opposite corner. Use the index finger of your right hand to open the mouth by pressing down on the lower teeth. As the cat opens its mouth, use the thumb and middle fingers of your left hand to compress the lips inward. This keeps the mouth open. Use a forceps or tweezer to place the pill deep into the animal's mouth (see Figure 42, page 180). As an alternative, drop the tablet deep into the open mouth. Use the eraser end of a pencil to tap the pill, or tap the back of the cat's throat; this causes the cat to swallow, and the medication goes down (see Figure 43, page 180). It is important to close the mouth quickly as the pencil is withdrawn. Hold the mouth closed and tap the cat briskly under the chin. Again, when the cat licks its nose, you will know that it has swallowed the medication.

Cats are especially suspicious of medication placed in their food. Even if you crush the tablet before mixing it with the food, you will not fool most cats—unless the medication is completely tasteless. However, both dogs and cats like brewer's yeast, cheese, and strong fish oil or chicken fat as flavoring agents; try adding one of these to the food when you want an especially tempting disguise.

GIVING LIQUID MEDICATION TO DOGS AND CATS

Cats and small dogs can be given 1 to 3 teaspoons of liquid medication at one dosing; large dogs may take 1 to 3 ounces without difficulty. It is best to measure the medication into a small prescription bottle or a liquid dosing vial, which has handy calibrations on the sides. These bottles or vials efficiently get the medi-

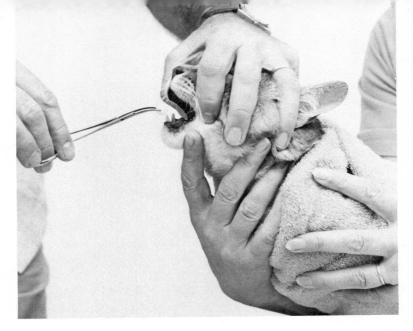

FIGURE 42. *Pilling a cat.* Secure the cat in a towel. Open the animal's mouth and use a forceps to drop the tablet deep into the throat.

FIGURE 43. *Alternate method of pilling a cat.* As an alternative, drop the tablet into the open mouth and use a pencil (eraser end) to tap the back of the throat. This stimulates the swallowing reflex. When the patient licks its nose, it has swallowed the medication.

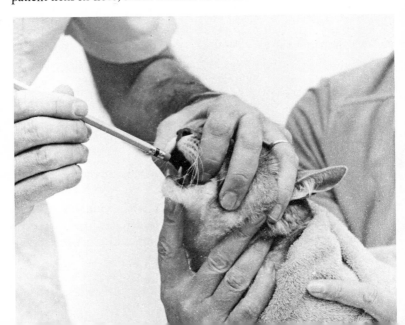

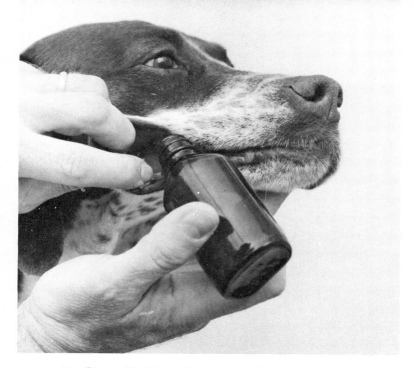

FIGURE 44. *Giving liquid medication to a dog.* Do not use a spoon. Put the prescribed amount of medicine in a small bottle. Pull out the corner of the lip to form a pocket. Pour the medicine in, a little at a time. As the liquid flows into the mouth and the patient swallows, add more medicine to the pocket. Do not elevate the nose; this allows the liquid to enter the air passages. A cat may be medicated the same way, but it is more difficult.

cation into the patient's mouth. Do not use a spoon—it is an abomination and it will usually spill much of the medication.

Hold the patient so it cannot shake its head, elevate its nose very slightly, and deposit the medication in the cheek pouch at the corner of the mouth. You can enlarge this pouch by pulling out the corner of the lip. (See Figure 44.) It may be necessary to open the animal's jaws slightly so the liquid flows between the teeth. When the liquid reaches the back of the mouth, the patient will swallow automatically. Patience and a gentle approach are needed for success.

Topical Medications

APPLICATION TO THE EYES
OF DOGS AND CATS

Eye drops must be applied frequently, since they tend to wash out rapidly with tears.

Elevate the patient's head and apply one or two drops of medication to the inner corner of the animal's eye. Liquid eye medication usually comes in a dropper bottle. If it does not, use an eye dropper. *Never* allow the applicator to touch the eyeball itself. (See Figure 45.)

Eye ointment usually comes in a ⅛-ounce tube. The ointment

FIGURE 45. *Application of eye drops.*

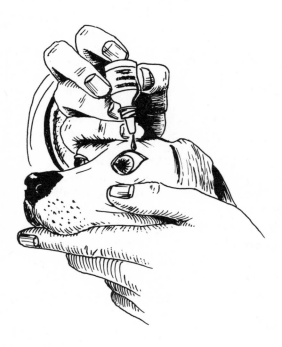

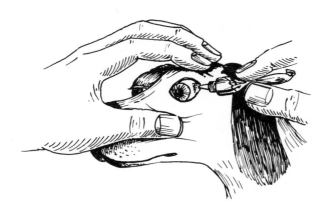

FIGURE 46. *Application of eye ointment.*

should be slightly warmer than room temperature so it will flow readily. Hold the patient's head firmly, open the eyelids, and pull the lower one slightly away from the eyeball. With the ointment tube, approach the eye from the rear of the head. Deposit a ⅛-inch-long strip of ointment on the lower lid lining near the outer corner of the eye (see Figure 46). The ointment will melt, and as the animal blinks, a film will spread over the eyeball.

APPLICATION TO THE NOSTRILS OF DOGS AND CATS

It is sometimes necessary to apply a watery solution of medication to an animal's nasal lining. Elevate the patient's head, with the nose pointing upward. Shield your pet's eyes so it cannot see what is happening. Without touching the nose with the dropper, apply several drops of the medication to the nasal passage. Gravity will cause the drops to run into the nose, and inhalation will spread them.

APPLICATION TO THE EARS
OF DOGS AND CATS

You will rarely apply powders and watery solutions to a pet's ears. However, you will be very likely to use ointments and oily solutions in the event of infection, inflammation, or parasites. Clean the ears with cotton pledgets dampened with alcohol. Then hold an ear flap up over the head and deposit a few drops of solution or an inch-long strip of ointment deep into the ear canal. Massage the base of the ear canal gently from the outside to spread the medication. It is important to get a film of the medication on the skin that lines the ear canal. Following the treatment the patient may shake its head a few times. This is not important.

APPLICATION TO THE SKIN
OF DOGS AND CATS

Use shampoos to wash noxious material from the surface of the skin. Some contain medication, but the effect lasts only as long as the shampoo is in contact with the skin. Leave the lather on for *at least* 10 to 15 minutes to provide *any* benefit.

To shampoo a dog, place it in a tub and put cotton into its ears and drops of cod-liver oil or a bland ointment into its eyes. Wet the coat thoroughly. Apply the shampoo along the back and work up a good lather. Rub well for 10 to 15 minutes and rinse thoroughly until the rinse water is clear. If it is not clear, repeat the shampoo.

A cat is usually more difficult to bathe, but it may be more tolerant of the procedures described above for dogs if you place it on a wire window screen and angle the screen in the tub. The cat will grip the screen with its claws and will then usually allow you to hold it in place for the shampoo. Bathe a cat only when it is essential—e.g., to remove toxic or greasy substances.

After the bath, dry the animal with a towel and/or blow dryer and comb the coat thoroughly. Some animals object to the noise of a dryer, but with patience you can train them to accept this—especially if you do so when they are young. As an alternative, confine the animal in a small shipping crate and direct the stream of warm air into the crate.

Use wet soaks for some skin inflammations and infections. To soak a foot, pour the solution into a large tomato or vegetable can and place the animal's foot into the can for the necessary amount of time. Only a small amount of fluid is needed, and the can's high sides prevent spilling. To soak areas of skin on the patient's body, dip a cloth in the solution and "sop" the area thoroughly. Then place the wet cloth over the affected skin for 10 to 15 minutes. Allow the skin to dry naturally. You can repeat these soaking procedures every three or four hours. Examples of soaking solutions include salt and water, chlorine solution, and Domeboro solution (see page 254).

Skin medication should be placed *on the skin*—not on the hair. To apply ointments and lotions, you will have to remove the hair in the affected areas by clipping or shaving it.

Lotions, such as calamine lotion, are fine suspensions of powder and water. After the water evaporates, a fine film of soothing powder is left on the skin. You will usually need to apply lotions several times daily; use cotton pledgets or your fingertips.

Shake medicated powder onto the skin to dry it and to make it slippery where skin chafes against skin. BFI powder is an example of a drying and healing powder. It is usually applied *sparingly* several times daily. You may also use powders to control fleas, lice, and ticks. In these cases, rub the hair the wrong way and apply the powder as the hair bristles up. This allows the powder to penetrate to the skin and adhere better. After such a dusting, wrap a dog or cat in a blanket or towel for a few minutes to improve the contact with parasites—and thus the kill.

Insect sprays (used to kill fleas and lice) and moisturizing sprays (such as AlphaKeri) are applied in much the same way as insecticidal powders. Spray them on from a distance of 12 to 15 inches and then gently rub them into the coat with your hands. These sprays give a nice shine to the coat and are often lightly perfumed.

Ointments are greasy medications with active ingredients that need to be in contact with the skin for a prolonged period. They are used to carry antibiotics, healing agents, and cortisonelike agents to the skin and to help retain moisture or soften dried, hard skin. Ointments should not be applied to the hair, but only to the skin surface. Shave or clip the hair away. Only a thin film of ointment is needed. You simply waste the medication if you apply an excess, since only the medication in contact with the skin will be effective.

27.

Taking the Temperature, Pulse, and Respiration

The temperature, pulse, and respiration rate (TPR) are vital signs, and they are important in determining your pet's reaction to many disorders. The animal's rectal temperature is a measure of its internal body heat. The pulse is the number of heartbeats per minute. The respiration (breathing) rate is the number of inspirations/expirations per minute. They are especially significant in cases of infection, heat or cold, injury, shock or stress, pregnancy, systemic acidity, lung disease, and hemorrhage. They are markedly affected by excitement, too; so to get really valid readings, you must check the vital signs when the patient is as relaxed as possible. They also vary with age, size, metabolic rate, time of day, and other normal factors. Therefore, an animal does not have an absolute "normal" single value for TPR; these values tend to fall into normal *ranges* (see page 258). It is a good idea to learn the normal range for *your* pet. If the animal becomes ill, you should look for abnormal trends by taking readings several times daily.

The Rectal Temperature

Always take an animal's temperature *rectally,* using a rectal thermometer. (Do *not* use an oral thermometer to take a rectal temperature. The bulb of mercury is long and thin and can easily break.) Rectal thermometers have a mercury column sealed in a glass capillary tube. A constriction near the bulb keeps the mercury from falling below its highest reading. Thus, before you use a thermometer, always shake it firmly until the column of mercury is just above the bulb (at about 96° F./36° C.).

To take the temperature, place the dog or cat on a table and confine it firmly in your arms (see Figure 47). Two people are usually needed for this procedure: one to restrain the animal and the other to take the temperature. Lubricate the thermometer bulb with soap or petroleum jelly. Grasp the patient's tail and elevate it slightly. Insert the thermometer through the anus with a gentle twisting motion until about half of its length is within the rectum. A cat may offer slight sphincter resistance, but persistent gentle pressure usually produces the necessary anal relaxation. Leave the

FIGURE 47. *Taking a temperature.* Shake the thermometer down to 96° F. (36° C.). Moisten the end with soapy water. Grasp the tail and elevate it slightly. Rotate the thermometer slightly as you press it through the anus.

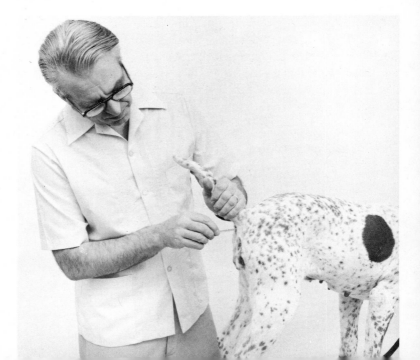

thermometer in place for *at least* 3 minutes. The thermometer and tail can be held together. *Do not* relax your grasp on the thermometer!

Remove the thermometer and wipe it off with cotton or a tissue. Then rotate the thermometer back and forth at eye level until the column of mercury is clearly visible. Read the number at the end of the mercury. Each small line between the numbers represents two-tenths of a degree. Record the results and if the illness is serious, repeat three or four times daily in order to obtain a true picture of temperature fluctuations. If you need to call your veterinarian, he will find this information exceedingly helpful.

Never wash a thermometer in hot water or expose it to high temperatures. Carefully clean it with soap and cool water, then rinse it, wipe it with rubbing alcohol, and store it in its plastic case for protection.

The normal temperature range for dogs is approximately 100° to 103° F. (101.5° F.) or 38° to 39° C.

The normal temperature range for cats is approximately 100° to 103° F. (101° F.) or 38° to 39° C.

The Pulse

To take the pulse of a dog or cat, press the index and middle fingers against the inside of the animal's hind leg, just below the point where it joins the body. A large artery (the femoral artery) crosses the thigh bone there, and in a normal dog or cat, you can easily feel the pulse. (See Figure 48, page 190.) There are other places where you can feel pulse—in fact, you may try any area where an artery is near the surface. In dogs and cats these areas are the underside of the tail near the body, and the rear (flexor) surface of the wrist joint on the front leg. However, when the animal is in shock, the pulse may be harder to find in these areas than at the rear leg. You can usually palpate the pulse while you are taking the animal's temperature. Once you locate the pulse, you should count it for at least 60 seconds.

If you only want to record the rate—and not the force—of the

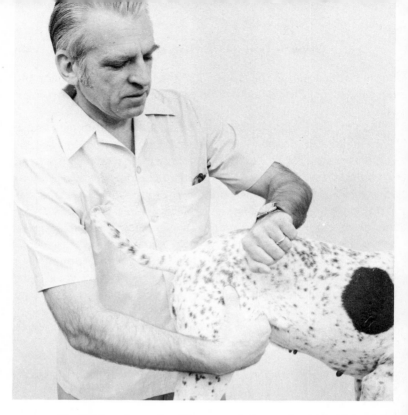

FIGURE 48. *Taking the pulse.* Use your index and middle fingers to feel the large artery running down the *inside* of the hind leg. Feel for it just below the point where the leg joins the body.

pulse, you can usually see the heart beating or feel it beating on the lower third of the chest just behind the elbow—especially on the left side of the chest (see Figure 2, page 16).

Many of the factors that increase the rectal temperature also increase the pulse. For the first-aider, the pulse is of special value in evaluating shock (see page 38). A fast pulse rate is characteristic of shock; a weak pulse or one that can hardly be felt is a serious sign. Dogs have a normal pulse irregularity. Ask your veterinarian to explain this to you. A cat's pulse is often so rapid that it may be difficult to count.

The normal pulse-rate range for a dog is 80 to 140 per minute; the normal range for a cat is 110 to 180 per minute.

The Respiration (Breathing) Rate

Always try to count the breathing rate when the animal is at rest. Excitement, heat, and exercise will markedly increase the rate, and although dogs and cats normally breathe only through their noses, they mouth-breathe as the rate increases. When the rate is rapid, they are said to "pant." Panting is a cooling mechanism. Air passes over the tongue and the mouth lining, which are richly supplied with blood. This helps to cool the blood and control body temperature. Panting is necessary, since dogs and cats do not perspire.

To determine the rate of breathing, count only the expirations (ribs contract and air goes out) *or* the inspirations (ribs expand and air goes in), but not both.

An animal will breathe rapidly if it is in shock or if it needs air or oxygen. Lung disease or an obstruction in the air passages will make the breathing difficult and labored. Try to notice if the patient has most of its difficulty breathing in or breathing out. Very deep respirations indicate a real air hunger or need for oxygen; shallow respirations indicate weakness or chest pain (as with pleurisy). Very irregular breathing, alternating from deep to shallow and then sighing, is a serious sign.

The normal respiratory-rate range for a dog is 10 to 30 per minute; the normal range for a cat is 20 to 30 per minute.

28.

Inducing Vomiting

Dogs and cats have the ability to vomit easily—in fact, almost at will. This is a protective mechanism that rids the stomach of poisonous or noxious substances or unloads an overstuffed stomach (a result of gluttonous eating). Food stays in the stomach for various lengths of time, depending on its composition. Large chunks of fatty substances may remain for up to 8 or 9 hours, while fine particles of carbohydrate or protein material may pass out of the stomach within an hour or two. A foreign object may remain for a very long time. By giving an emetic (a drug that causes vomiting) early in the course of a problem, the stomach can be cleared of abnormal or toxic substances before they are absorbed or cause serious complications. Do *not* give an emetic if a corrosive chemical or a sharp object has been ingested, if the patient is unconscious, or if there is an obstruction of the throat or esophagus.

When to Induce Vomiting to Empty the Stomach

1. The dog or cat has very recently eaten a noncorrosive poisonous material that has not had time to be absorbed.
2. The animal has swallowed a soft or blunt object, such as a piece of cloth, a sock, powder puff, or piece of blanket; small pieces of stone or gravel; powders; or round foreign objects.
3. The animal has overeaten or has eaten difficult-to-digest food, such as excessive grease, garbage, bird or cow feed, or uncooked grains.

Procedure

1. Administer 1 to 2 teaspoons of hydrogen peroxide (medicinal) by mouth to dogs; 1 teaspoon to cats. Repeat the dose every 10 to 15 minutes until the patient vomits. Mild peroxide is safe, readily available, and very effective. Most pets vomit within a few minutes after the first or second dose.

2. As an alternative for dogs only, give 1 tablespoonful of very concentrated salt solution (mix 1 tablespoon salt with 1 cup water) by mouth. However, this solution is not as effective as hydrogen peroxide. Another method for dogs is to place ½ teaspoon of dry salt in the rear of the animal's throat. These salt emetics usually work better if the dog is made to drink a large quantity of water (1 to 8 ounces) afterward.

3. If these methods fail, your veterinarian can give an injection of a potent drug that will make a dog vomit promptly.

Remember, any action necessary to make a dog or cat vomit implies some serious problem. Call or visit your veterinarian to clear any questions, and make sure your pet has follow-up care if necessary. If you think that poison was involved, save some of the vomited material and take it with you to your veterinarian. Examine the vomitus carefully so you can describe its color, consistency, and odor and can report the presence of any blood or mucus.

If veterinary aid is not immediately available, refer to pages 43 and 53–67 for directions on handling poisonings.

29.

Giving an Enema

An enema is a fluid preparation that is injected through the anus into the rectum and lower colon. It is usually given to empty the lower bowel and relieve constipation, to evacuate the rectum before surgery or whelping, or to remove impacted fecal material or a smooth foreign body. After a cleansing enema, certain medications or nutrient materials such as sugar and salts can be injected into the rectum and retained for absorption. Your veterinarian may also use an enema incorporating an X-ray opaque substance that outlines the lower bowel for diagnostic X-ray studies. In this book we are concerned only with the enema used to cleanse the bowel of undesirable materials.

Procedure

1. Prepare the patient. Clip the hair away from the anus (if necessary) and apply a film of petroleum jelly or soap solution to lubricate the anal region.

2. Muzzle the animal if it appears to be snappy or apprehensive about being handled.

3. Confine the patient to a large tub (bathtub) or to a restricted grassy yard area if there is one available.

4. Hold the animal firmly in a standing position. Two people will be needed for any dog or cat.

5. Give Colace capsules orally as preparation for an enema, or add Colace to the enema water. This product helps water penetrate hard, dry feces and produces a beneficial softening effect.

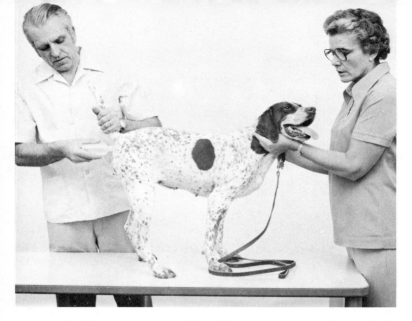

FIGURE 49. *Giving an enema.* The Fleet enema comes in a plastic bottle with a long nozzle. Insert the nozzle through the anus as you would a rectal thermometer. Squeeze the bottle slowly to inject its contents into the rectum. Hold the patient firmly during the enema. When all the fluid has been injected, quickly release the animal in an appropriate "toilet area."

DOGS

6. Use a Fleet enema. This is a 4-ounce plastic bottle with an attached nozzle, manufactured for commercial sales by Fleet, and it is one of the handiest ways to give an enema to a dog. The Fleet saline enema solution works effectively. You can buy it at any pharmacy.

Insert the lubricated nozzle through the anus and gently inject 1 to 4 ounces of the solution (warmed to body temperature) into the rectum. (See Figure 49.) Use no more than 1 ounce for toy breeds, 2 ounces for terriers (20 to 30 pounds) and 3 to 4 ounces for dogs larger than 30 pounds. Following injection, hold the nozzle in place for a minute or two. Then release the patient. It will usually strain and return a spray of enema fluid mixed with particles of feces. The process can be repeated once or twice at 20-minute intervals. Remove the feces from the tub and clean the whole area thoroughly after you have finished the enema.

7. As an alternative, make your own enema solution. A solution of Ivory soap or gentle Castile soap and warm water (1 ounce of liquid soap to 1 quart of water) may be used instead of the prepackaged saline solution. Another enema solution is 1 ounce of glycerine to 3 ounces of water. Pour *one* of these solutions into an elevated funnel or enema can attached to a soft rubber tube. Lubricate the end of the tube and insert it into the patient's rectum. This method requires at least two people: one or more to restrain the patient and one to hold the tube in place as the gravity-fed solution enters the patient. Administer the solution slowly and gently. Give only 4 ounces to small canine breeds, up to 1 pint to spaniel-sized dogs, and up to 1 quart to large breeds. Repeat the enema, in a smilar amount, once, 1 hour later, if necessary.

CATS

8. Restrain a cat for an enema by wrapping it in a heavy blanket, with just its rear quarters exposed. Cats in particular may resent the indignity of an enema, and they are especially prone to develop signs of shock from too vigorous a procedure.

The enema solution preferred for cats is Ivory soap or gentle Castile soap and warm water (1 ounce of liquid soap to 1 quart of water). Inject 3 to 4 ounces only. The process will be messy; so proper facilities for easy cleanup afterward are essential.

DOGS AND CATS

9. For mild constipation, try suppositories. These are often just as effective as enemas. You can make them from pencil-shaped slivers of a cake of soap or purchase pediatric glycerine suppositories from a pharmacy.

Insert the suppository into the anus and leave it in place. Follow the manufacturer's directions carefully.

10. Taking a pet's temperature with a rectal thermometer will often serve to stimulate a bowel movement.

11. When mild constipation appears to be a problem, add mineral oil (1 to 6 teaspoons) to the pet's food once a day for several days. Follow with an enema if necessary.

12. An enema can be an exhausting procedure for your pet. This is especially true for cats. Gentleness and patience are mandatory. If you have problems, it is best to seek veterinary help.

III.

MISCELLANEOUS PROBLEM SOLVING

30.

Selecting a Veterinarian

Like all medical professionals, veterinarians must undergo many years of arduous schooling. They must then pass a rigorous state licensing examination in order to practice veterinary medicine. However, once licensed, each doctor's future development varies considerably. Some veterinarians remain generalists, treating all kinds of problems in several species of animals. Some restrict their interests to one or two species, while others narrow their goals to a specialty practice (such as surgery, dermatology, or ophthalmology). Specialists are relatively new to veterinary medicine and are most often found in teaching hospitals or large practices in an urban area. Veterinarians often work together for the best interest of their patients; so don't be surprised if yours refers you to a colleague who has more expertise or more complete facilities for handling your pet's specific problem. Although this type of treatment will be more expensive, referral is a reflection of your veterinarian's concern for your pet.

There are several ways to get recommendations concerning the veterinary service in your area. Get a variety of opinions by asking neighbors, other pet owners, breeders, and members of a kennel club, or call the local Veterinary Society. Use the following guidelines to help find the veterinarian that will best meet your needs.

In selecting someone to care for your pet's medical problems, he or she should

1. Be a licensed veterinarian.

2. Have a clean, modern, well-kept facility to treat your species of pet. The location should be convenient to you.

3. Enjoy caring for your species of pet.

4. Provide coverage for emergencies. (Record the data needed to get help in the front of this book.)

In addition, the following items may indicate a potential for superior care.

1. The hospital provides complete laboratory, surgical, and radiological services on the premises.

2. The hospital has been inspected and listed as approved by a state or national organization. However, some excellent hospitals have not been approved, since this is a new, voluntary program.

3. The professional staff keep up with medical advances by frequent attendance of continuing-education courses.

4. The individual veterinarian is board-certified in a specialty area (such as internal medicine or surgery). Almost all veterinarians belong to their local and national professional associations.

Some personal items should enter into your decision.

1. Is your veterinarian available to you when your pet has a problem?

2. Are your personal concerns satisfied?

3. Does the personality of your veterinarian mesh with yours?

4. Are the professional charges acceptable to you?

If you can respond favorably to most of the above criteria, you have found your veterinarian. Trust him or her and follow the advice carefully. However, don't expect the impossible. Remember that pets are relatively short-lived and that many diseases are incurable. In some cases, continued treatment may not be a kindness to you or to your pet. Your veterinarian can be a sympathetic source of strength and a good friend, too.

31.

Pet Foods

The pet food industry is a multimillion-dollar business that produces thousands of individual brands and types of food. The largest concerns spend fortunes on research and development, and the products labeled "complete and balanced" have sustained pets successfully through several generations. No amateur nutritionist can provide a diet comparable in balance, convenience, and economy by mixing ingredients at home.

Each commercial diet is designed for a single species. In some cases you can use a formula for more than one species, but you should do so on a temporary basis only. Dogs do quite well on some cat foods, but cats will not thrive on dog foods. Cats find dog food unpalatable, and the canine formulas are too low in calories, protein, and fat to meet feline needs. (For more details consult the tables of nutrient requirements, pages 262–263, and the list of references at the end of the book, page 265.)

The array of colored cans and pet-food packages on supermarket shelves can be terribly confusing to the pet owner. The following is a description of the types of food available, with comments on the advantages and disadvantages of each.

Dog Foods

Dog foods can provide complete balanced nutrition for your dog, or they can be incomplete "treat" or supplemental foods. There are three types, categorized according to moisture content—dry, moist, and soft-moist. Within each of these types, there are foods formulated to meet certain special needs of the changing life cycles of dogs. These major periods are the growing puppy, the pregnant and nursing mother, the obese pet, the senior citizen, and the average, vigorous adult house pet. Although progressive manufacturers are now marketing foods designed for specific life stages and conditions, the majority of complete dog foods are designed for maintenance of the average pet. The latter foods are generally quite adequate and with a little modification, are adaptable to other life stages and situations.

A satisfactory diet should keep your dog healthy, alert, and vigorous, with a glossy coat and bright eyes. It should produce normal stools and no evidence of digestive upsets.

Palatability (taste) is a great concern for most pet owners. If the pet doesn't eat the food, of course it will be of no benefit; but the fact that the pet eats eagerly does not necessarily mean the food has special merit. Palatability for many pets is determined by "mouth feel." Some dogs like dry, crunchy food, while others prefer to have the same food soaked so that it is moist or even soft and mushy. High levels of animal protein and animal fat make food appetizing, and some individual dogs like flavoring agents, such as garlic or onion salt. However, these last items may make your pet less acceptable as a household pet several hours later.

TYPES OF DOG FOODS

DRY DOG FOODS

Dry dog foods are marketed as meals, biscuits, kibbles, and expanded foods. They contain 8 to 10% moisture and approximately 1600 calories per pound. Dry foods keep well and are economical; so they are popular kennel foods. Biscuits do not provide balanced nutrition and should only be used as treats or training rewards. The other dry foods offer complete, balanced nutrition, and with water, they provide all that the average pet needs to stay healthy. Expanded foods are crunchy particles coated with fat. They are very light and bulky (a large bag is light in weight). Dry foods are the only type of ration that is well adapted to self-feeding (see page 211).

You may feed your dog dry foods exclusively—either completely dry or moistened with water to the consistency your pet prefers. Some owners add meat, cheese, canned food, or cooked table scraps to dry food to produce variety or to improve palatability. To retain the basic balance of the food, do not let these "other" ingredients exceed 25% of the total diet.

MOIST DOG FOODS

Moist foods may be fresh, frozen, or canned. Depending on the fat content, they contain 75 to 80% moisture and 500 to 600 calories per pound.

Without supplementation, all-meat products are poor nutrition—especially for growing puppies and pregnant bitches. (Digestive upsets or severe musculoskeletal deformities may develop, and puppy fatalities have been reported.) These products are highly palatable but very expensive. Small amounts may be added to balanced dry foods.

The canned products sold as balanced diets are supplemented with many ingredients to overcome the problems described above. The better foods are usually puddinglike mixtures of meat and meat by-products, vegetables, and cereals, with vitamins and minerals added as needed. These products are about 75% water and provide about 500 calories per pound. Most cans, however, are not a full pound (16 ounces). Although most appear to be the same size, the cans vary from 13 to 15½ ounces in weight, and the water content varies, too.

Some canned dog foods contain only meat, with vitamins and minerals added. Although these are technically balanced, they contain more protein than is necessary for most dogs, and they are particularly expensive. Some dogs have digestive upsets when fed these diets exclusively.

SOFT-MOIST (SEMI-MOIST) DOG FOODS

These products are sold in sealed plastic pouches. The food looks like hamburger patties or cubes of meat, and contains 30% moisture with about 1300 calories per pound. This relatively dense caloric formula makes the products desirable for puppies, pregnant bitches, and toy breeds. But because it is so rich and so palatable, your pet may gain weight from overeating. These products are easy to digest and convenient, and they keep well as long as the package remains sealed. Soft-moist foods are all balanced diets; you can add them to dry foods, as you wish. You can also mix them with milk or warm water to make a mush—a particularly good diet for very young puppies.

SPECIAL DIETS FOR DOGS

Your veterinarian may prescribe a special diet if your dog has a specific disease problem. He may recommend a specially formulated diet, a modified regular dog food, or a special product formulated and marketed commercially for a specific dietary need. This last item is expensive but very much worth the money. In most cases, these diets are necessary for only a short period of time (to reduce obesity or to correct digestive problems), but in some instances diet management may be a life-long necessity. These diets are not meant for routine feeding of normal, healthy pets.

SUPPLEMENTS AND SPECIAL FOODS

BONES

Bones probably produce more grief than pleasure for dogs. *Never* feed your pet small chicken or chop bones. They may splinter and lacerate the dog's mouth or become lodged in the digestive tract. You may give large knuckle or shank bones to a dog that is teething or if you want the dog to stimulate its gums and clean its teeth by gnawing. There is no doubt dogs enjoy bones, but hard biscuits or rawhide toys are probably as effective—and they are safer.

TABLE SCRAPS

Your leftovers are usually an excellent source of varied nutrients for dogs. Dogs digest cooked starches and carbohydrates well, and almost any table foods—such as dairy products, vegetables, potatoes, noodles, eggs, meat, or fish—will do. Avoid highly spiced foods, rich pastries, or exotic foods. Never give your dog alcoholic beverages, spoiled or tainted food, or garbage and raw starches.

EGGS

Eggs are the ideal protein for dogs. They provide perfectly balanced amino acids; and since *high quality* protein may be the deficient ingredient in pet foods, growing or pregnant dogs almost always benefit by a diet supplemented with eggs. Raw eggs, however, may be difficult to digest, and may even interfere with proper utilization of biotin (a vitamin). Try to feed your dog cooked eggs. Cheese and other dairy products are also excellent foods for dogs.

VITAMIN AND MINERAL SUPPLEMENTS

Vitamin and mineral supplements are rarely necessary and you should not give them routinely unless they are prescribed by your veterinarian. Feed a complete, balanced diet composed of many ingredients. This is the best way to provide the trace elements needed for good health.

Cat Foods

Cat foods are available in three major types—dry, moist, and semi-most—which are quite similar to dog foods in moisture content but quite different in composition. Cat foods usually contain higher percentages of protein and fat than dog foods.

TYPES OF CAT FOODS

DRY CAT FOODS

Dry cat food contains meat and vegetables, with about 9 to 10% moisture and about 30% protein and 8% fat. You can moisten this food to the desired consistency or serve it dry. Many owners leave unmoistened food in the food dish constantly so the cat can nibble as it wishes. This is ideal, since cats are frequent nibblers (as compared to dogs, which gulp their food rapidly and infrequently).

MOIST CAT FOODS

Moist cat food usually comes in cans, with about 75% moisture and the balance protein and fat. The small "treat" cans of variety foods are usually all-meat or all-fish. Tuna fish is often used in these packs. Although these products are extremely tasty and are excellent protein sources, they are not nutritionally balanced—so you should not feed them as the total diet. Some cats become "addicted" to exclusive diets of liver or tuna fish and will eat nothing else. Be certain the cat has a variety of types and brands of food.

Some canned cat foods are well-balanced, complete diets. They are labeled as such and usually packaged in larger cans than the all-meat or all-fish products. All these maintenance diets support adult cats adequately, but they may not be satisfactory for growing kittens or pregnant cats. The cans contain more than enough food for one cat for one day, and the balance should be stored under refrigeration. However, never feed this food cold or digestive disturbances may result. Warm the food to room temperature.

SEMI-MOIST CAT FOODS

Semi-moist cat foods are similar to those dog-food products that come in sealed plastic pouches. They contain about 27% protein and 7% fat, with about 35% water. They are highly palatable, provide complete, balanced nutrition, and are available in different flavors. Leave the food in the food dish all day for frequent nibbling or feed periodically as desired.

The discussion of special diets for dogs (see page 206) applies to cats also. Cats should *not* be fed dog foods, raw fish or pork, large amounts of liver, raw eggs, or any bones. They rarely require mineral and vitamin supplements. When and if needed, these medications should be prescribed by your veterinarian.

32.

Feeding Dogs and Cats

Feeding Your Dog

Feed your dog *like a dog*—not like a cat or a human. Dogs do well on a constant, unvarying formula diet through much of their life span. Modify the diet as they become diseased or develop unusual physiological needs—but otherwise dogs do well and are happy on foods that people would consider monotonous. However, the dietary needs of individual dogs may vary considerably. The requirements of a 2-pound Chihuahua are considerably different from those of a 140-pound St. Bernard. Small breeds need a dense caloric formula. These dogs need 40 to 50 calories per pound of body weight per day, and they must receive the nutrition in a small volume of food. Large breeds, on the other hand, need only 20 to 30 calories per pound per day, and since they can eat a large volume at one time, their food can have a less concentrated formula. In spite of these differences, most commercial dog foods adequately nourish all but the very unusual adult dog.

The pet owner who tries to compound his own dog food using only household ingredients faces a formidable task and, unless he or she is a trained nutritionist, will end up with an expensive and decidedly inferior product. Many pet owners spoil their dogs by giving them treats and table foods with high appetite appeal. Often, by refusing to eat a regular dog food, the dog "trains" its owners to provide exotic foods that may not be adequate nutritionally. Resist this ploy! Feeding snacks or treats also causes obesity. If you wish to use foods as training rewards, subtract the amount of the treats from your dog's daily ration.

The single key to successful dog feeding is to *feed only a complete, balanced diet*. It should be produced by a commercial company that has done research and made feeding trials through several generations of dogs to prove the diet is adequate for all life stages. The diet can be dry, soft-moist, moist, or combinations of these. Adhere to the balanced diets and you will not go far astray. Follow the manufacturer's feeding directions carefully.

Dry foods are least expensive. Moisten or not as the dog prefers, and feed to adults once daily. If you add cooked table scraps or meat to the dry food, these can comprise up to 25% of the total daily intake without upsetting the nutritional balance of the diet. One ounce of most dry foods will nourish 3 to 4 pounds of dog for one day. Dry, expanded dog foods are the ideal for self-feeding. About 90% of dogs can maintain an ideal weight by this method. The other 10% eat too much and become obese.

To self-feed, give the dog an adequate meal the first day and then place a large dish of expanded food in the usual feeding place. The dog will nibble frequently and over 24 hours eat what is needed. The food consumption will vary automatically with the amount of energy expended or with climatic changes. Keep the dish full by adding fresh food to the *bottom* of the dish as needed. This will rotate the food properly. Self-feeding is an excellent method for either house or kennel dogs. It is inexpensive, easy, saves waste, and eliminates begging and barking at feeding time. It is especially useful if you will be away for a day or two and must feed penned dogs. About 10% of dogs that are self-fed overeat and become obese. These dogs must be fed measured amounts of food at specific intervals.

Soft-moist dog food is a relatively new food concept, ideally suited for feeding finicky eaters and young puppies. (For young puppies, mix the food with milk or water to make a mush.) Soft-moist foods can also be added to dry foods, or fed once or twice daily, as the only source of food. One ounce of this sealed-in-plastic food provides an adequate diet for 2 to 3 pounds of dog for one day.

Moist or canned foods should only be fed exclusively if they provide complete and balanced nutrition. One ounce of these products provides nutrition for about one pound of dog for one day. Diets of moist foods alone may upset some dogs' digestive systems; therefore, it is wise to use them in combination with a dry food. Canned foods are expensive but highly palatable. Do not use them for self-feeding, since they dry out and spoil. Also, because of their palatability, they encourage dogs to overeat. Feed your dog moist food once or twice daily at a regular meal time. Refrigerate any food left in the can and always warm the leftover portion to room temperature before serving.

The new commercial foods designed for special needs of the different life stages and conditions of a dog's life have much to offer. Ask your veterinarian if they fit your pet's needs.

Frequency of feeding depends on several factors. Self-feeding is the most frequent rate, while once-a-day feeding is adequate for most adult dogs. There is nothing wrong with occasionally skipping a day's feeding. In nature, dogs were hunters and when they were unsuccessful, they became accustomed to fasting. On the other hand, when they had food, they would bolt it down in large gulps. Many of our pets still eat rapidly and swallow large chunks of food. This is actually desirable since large pieces of food remain in the stomach longer and are thus more completely digested than finely ground particles, which may pass through the stomach too rapidly.

For more details about feeding, see pages 262–264 in the appendix and write for *Nutritional Requirements of Dogs,* Committee on Animal Nutrition, Agricultural Board, National Academy of Sciences, National Research Council, Washington, D.C.

Like all animals, dogs require fresh, pure water. Keep it available at all times. Discourage drinking from a toilet bowl or other unsanitary source. The amount of water dogs consume varies according to the type of food they eat (dry food creates a need for more water), the amount of exercise they get (more active dogs need more water), and the environmental temperature (high temperatures make dogs thirstier). Most dogs drink the largest percentage of their daily water shortly after being fed. If your dog drinks an excessive amount of water, this could be a sign of illness. See your veterinarian for a check-up.

The following are common *mistaken* beliefs:

1. Milk causes worms.
2. Garlic is a cure for worms.
3. Dogs and cats need milk all their lives.
4. Dogs need all-meat diets, and cereal is bad for them.
5. All dogs need high-protein diets.
6. High-protein diets cause kidney or liver disease.
7. Rich foods are good for older pets.
8. Canned (moist) or soft-moist foods are superior to dry foods.
9. Finicky eaters cannot be trained to accept different foods (that may be better balanced).
10. Dogs need or should have bones to chew.
11. Food costs are proportional to nutritional value.
12. Palatability of food is an indication of its nutritional value.

Feeding Your Cat

Feed your cat *like a cat*—not like a dog or a human. Cats like variety, and they are nibblers, happy to snack at frequent intervals. They are also finicky, and after carefully sniffing at your latest gourmet offering, they may walk away in complete disdain. On the other hand, cats easily become addicted to one food—especially such items as liver, fresh meat, or tuna fish. None of these is an adequate exclusive diet for cats. Cats are usually sensible about managing the amount of food they eat, and very few overeat to the extent that they become obese. If they do, suspect your feeding program or look for a psychological disturbance. Then eliminate the cause.

In nature cats usually are expert hunters, and they balance their diets by catching and eating every morsel of their prey. They catch all kinds of small rodents, birds, lizards, and snakes and often proudly bring them home to demonstrate their hunting prowess.

Eating wild prey exposes your cat to several disease states—especially toxoplasmosis and internal parasites—and you should prevent this habit. The only way to stop the hunting habit in a cat is to keep it confined. However, you can discourage the habit by "belling the cat" or having it declawed. Many veterinarians recommend removing the front claws (toenails). It is a simple procedure and it prevents indoor cats from scratching furniture (or people). It also makes the cat less able to fight and hunt, but surprisingly, a declawed cat can still easily climb a tree, especially if pursued by an aggressive dog.

Do not feed cats table foods or foods that are cold. The best method is to leave dry or soft-moist cat food available to your pet at all times. Place an amount that is slightly more than is needed for 24 hours in a dish and replenish daily. Rotate the food by adding the fresh food to the *bottom* of the dish. This prevents food from being left in the bottom of the dish for several days. This method is effective, as cats enjoy nibbling.

Some cat owners like to expand and supplement the above system by feeding the cat a different food as a "meal" once or twice daily. These feedings may consist of canned cat food, canned treats, liver or fish, fresh meat, or cottage cheese. A cat will usually relish such a meal, and under this system, will eat correspondingly less of the constantly available dry or soft-moist foods.

The amount of food a cat needs varies, depending on growth, physical activity, pregnancy, metabolic rate, and digestive efficiency. You must tailor the amounts to your own cat's needs. Most adult cats weigh between 6 and 10 pounds. Generally either 2 to 3 ounces of dry food, 2 to 4 ounces of soft-moist food, or 5 to 8 ounces of canned food will provide maintenance requirements. However, kittens and pregnant cats require much more than this. The best maintenance guide is to feed your cat an amount adequate to maintain a constant and ideal body weight. The above quantities are rough guides. Read and carefully follow feeding advice on the cat-food package or can. Feed a variety of foods.

Like all animals, cats require fresh, pure water. The amount they drink depends on the kind of food they are fed. If they are fed canned food (70% water) they will drink much less than if they are fed dry food (8% water). Always keep fresh water available. Do not allow your cat to drink from the toilet bowl, flower dish, fish tank, or other unsanitary source. Some cats favor milk. However, milk should be considered a food, not a source of water. Offer milk only after the cat has eaten its solid food. A surprising number of cats develop diarrhea and digestive upsets from milk. If you suspect this, avoid feeding milk or other dairy products to your cat.

33.

Internal Parasites (Worms)

Internal parasites are organisms that inhabit internal organs of the body, such as the digestive tract, liver, lungs, and muscles. There are several kinds of internal parasites that affect dogs, cats, and other pet animals. Each presents a specific problem, and each requires a different medication and sanitation practice for effective control. It is impossible to simply go to the pharmacy and purchase a medicine to safely and effectively worm a dog. A more precise diagnosis is needed. Many pet owners have the mistaken idea that almost any pet disease is due to "worms," and they try a worm medication first. *Never* do this, as it often worsens an already serious illness. All worm medicines are poisons—meant to poison the worm but not the patient. There are many safe and effective worm medications; however, if you use the wrong drug, give an incorrect dosage, or worm when the patient is debilitated with another disease, you may poison your pet. Always get an accurate diagnosis and a prescription for correct medication from your veterinarian.

The problem of internal parasites varies markedly from area to area. Parasites tend to thrive in moist, warm climates; so they are especially troublesome in the southeastern United States. They do not thrive as well in cold northern climates. However, it is best not to make generalizations. Get specific advice for your pet in your locality.

The following information is general background data about some common parasites. But again—seek specific advice from your veterinarian.

Types of Worms

ROUNDWORMS (ASCARIDS)

These worms have a direct life cycle (i.e., they are spread directly from dog to dog) and are most serious as a health hazard to young puppies and kittens. Periodic worming is mandatory for these young pets. As your pet matures, it usually develops a tolerance to the worms, and the few that remain cause no problem. It is impossible to completely eradicate them, and contrary to popular opinion, they do not cause pain and do not need monthly treatment for life.

Puppies and kittens with roundworms may be thin and pot-bellied and have hiccups, chronic diarrhea, and occasional vomiting. Repeat worm medication frequently during the early weeks of life and thereafter as prescribed. Most of these medications are inexpensive and safe.

HOOKWORMS

Hookworms also have a direct life cycle, but they can infect and produce illness in dogs of all ages, especially those kept in unsanitary conditions. The immature worms invade the skin or are ingested and can cause real problems in kennel or crowded conditions. The same dog can reinfect itself. Hookworms are especially lethal to pets 2 to 3 weeks old. They cause a severe, bloody diarrhea, so that the animal is not only thin, weak, and malnourished but severely anemic. Hookworms rarely affect cats.

Medications for the parasites must be used at the proper time and dosage and with great care. Interrupting the life cycle of the parasite is as important as the medication itself. Keep the animal and its environment scrupulously clean and remove feces from the animal's play area often. Pave or treat a run surface with salt or borax to help kill the infective stage of the parasite. (Caution: these chemicals may kill grass and trees in the area treated.) Some dogs may need periodic stool examinations and wormings throughout their entire life span to adequately control hookworms.

WHIPWORMS

Whipworms also have a direct life cycle, and their eggs may remain in the ground, as a source of infection, for several years. The parasite only affects dogs—usually older puppies or mature dogs. Whipworms are acquired when dogs are confined to an area where infected dogs were previously housed. The parasites live in the dog's lower intestinal tract. Symptoms include intermittent diarrhea, weight loss, anemia, and generally poor health. The stool that is passed may be very soft and usually contains mucus. Examine the stool frequently to establish the diagnosis. Treat with oral medication for several days. Repeat the therapy once or twice at intervals of several months. Since reinfection is typical, frequent fecal examinations are necessary to identify and control the parasite. As with hookworms, control depends on breaking the life cycle of the parasite by improving hygiene and sanitary conditions.

STRONGYLOIDES

Strongyloides is a very small parasite that lives in the upper part of the intestinal tract of infected dogs. Part of the life cycle is spent in a form that is free-living, outside the dog. This parasite is one of the few that might infect several species including man, so it is a public-health hazard. Use caution in handling infected dogs.

Strongyloides infections are most common in kenneled dogs or those housed in unsanitary conditions. Affected dogs are usually mature. Symptoms include watery diarrhea, which may contain blood; loss of weight; depression; and poor appetite.

The infection used to be considered almost incurable, but effective treatment is now available. It is important to have regular monthly fecal examinations for one year after the treatment has been completed, to identify relapses or reinfection.

TAPEWORMS

These worms are intestinal parasites that have an indirect life cycle. This means that one stage of their life must pass through an intermediate host—one other than your pet. The dog or cat can only be infected by ingesting the form of the parasite that is contained in the intermediate host. If the host is eliminated or separated from the dog or cat, tapeworm infection is impossible. Pets that ingest fleas, rodents (mice, rabbits), or infected fish, raw pork, or beef may acquire tapeworms. Careful inspection and thorough cooking of meat largely remove the latter source of infection. The main thrust of tapeworm control in pets involves elimination of fleas and rodents—sometimes a difficult task.

Oral medication to remove tapeworms present in the intestinal tract is the second facet of control. Tapeworm medications are expensive but effective when used properly. You may have to repeat the treatment periodically because the pet may be reinfected. It is a peculiar fact that of a group of dogs housed together, only one (or several) may be heavily infested.

Tapeworms rarely cause severe disease states. They usually affect relatively mature animals. Symptoms include loss of weight and mild diarrhea. The usual sign is the presence of small segments of tapeworms in the stool. These segments may be found in a dried state, in the pet's bedding or attached to the hair around the anus or under the tail. This is mainly an aesthetic—not a medical—problem.

HEARTWORMS

Heartworms inhabit the blood and tissues. They may produce severe damage to the heart, lungs, and liver—and may even cause death. They affect adult dogs. Treatment has considerable risk in severe cases but is not serious in mild cases. Try to protect your dog from exposure or use prophylactic measures to avoid infection. Cats rarely have heartworms.

Heartworms require a mosquito as an intermediate host and so, have an indirect life cycle. A mosquito withdraws blood from an infected dog and in the process ingests immature forms of the heartworm. These must mature in the mosquito for two weeks before they can infect dogs. When a mosquito bites a dog at this later time, it injects the infective larvae (immature heartworms) into the dog. These immature forms can then continue their growth cycle and develop into adults. They pass through the tissues and blood vessels and lodge in the heart, where they live for the balance of their lives—up to 5 years. If very numerous, they interfere with heart function. When the adult worms die, they may be passed along to the lungs, where they cause more problems.

Heartworms are common in the southern and eastern United States, but there are increasing numbers in other areas that have a heavy mosquito population. To control heartworms, you must prevent your dog from being bitten by mosquitos. Keep it indoors during evenings or dark days when mosquitos are active, keep it in screened quarters, or use local spraying and area mosquito control.

An additional aid is available. When your pet has had a blood test and you are sure it is free of heartworms, you can give a prophylactic medication during the mosquito season. The drug, diethylcarbamazine, is sold under several trade names. In areas with a mosquito season, you *must* give it *daily,* starting 30 days before the mosquito season and continuing for 60 days after it. For areas that have a year-round mosquito season, the drug must be given daily all year.

Dogs with heartworms receive injected medication for the adult worms. This is followed by a period of absolute rest while the dead worms are being dissolved and eliminated by the body. A second drug is then given to eliminate the immature parasites in the tissues. Following this, the preventive medication described above can be started.

Some dogs with heartworms do not show any symptoms but are a source of infection for other dogs. Pets with severe infections may be anemic, have a chronic cough, lose weight, and have poor stamina. The disease can be serious, but with proper care, it can be prevented or successfully treated.

34.

External Parasites
(Fleas, Lice, Ticks, and Mange Mites)

External parasites are insectlike organisms that live on or just under the surface of the skin for all or part of their life cycles. External parasites are a major cause of skin problems in dogs and cats. They cause much itching and discomfort and may spread infections and other diseases. Most external parasites will attack many species of animals. Mange mites, however, are an exception, as they usually are quite host-specific. Some parasites spend all or most of their time *on* their host, while others spend most of their life cycle *off* their host, only attaching themselves to the animal for short feeding periods. Understanding the cycles is important for effective treatment and control.

Insecticides are used to treat external parasites. These are toxic agents, which must be used with care. Eliminating the parasite on the premises (rather than on the patient) is always safer and often more effective. Medications applied to the animal must be tailored to the individual's specific needs. Since new drugs are constantly being developed, the comments here concern *general* control measures.

Types of Parasites

FLEAS

Fleas are small, brown wingless insects with laterally compressed bodies. They have long powerful legs that enable them to jump and travel easily and rapidly. The adults are blood-suckers that spend only part of their lives on the host; the eggs and immature forms are found mostly on the premises frequented by the host (your pet). The life cycle of the flea can be as short as three weeks or as long as two years, depending on environmental temperatures and humidity. Fleas thrive in moist, warm areas; they cannot survive in climates of low humidity or in altitudes of more than about 6000 feet. In cold weather the adults die, but the eggs and immature forms survive to produce adult fleas when the weather moderates.

Fleas may produce a minor effect with their bite in the skin, but they also produce a more severe generalized allergic reaction. They may cause so much scratching and self-mutilation that many other skin problems are worsened. Most of the lesions from fleas are noticed on the back or neck, especially on the back just in front of the tail. You can diagnose fleas by finding either the adult flea or deposits of flea excrement (dark, gritty particles) in the pet's hair. Because they contain much blood, these particles turn reddish brown when moistened and smeared on white paper.

Flea control entails two principles: treatment of the host animal and—even more important—treatment of the premises. Dogs and cats can be sprayed or dusted with preparations containing carbaryl, pyrethrins, or other insecticides. Dogs can be "dipped" with several products that are safe and effective. Cats, on the other hand, need special care. Many insecticides may poison them. In all cases, follow manufacturers' directions explicitly. When applying a spray or powder, rub the hair "the wrong way" as you sprinkle or spray the dust into the hair; this will ensure penetration and adherence beneath the coat. Wrap your pet in a towel for a few minutes —this will hold in the fleas and improve the kill. Repeat this treatment several times a week. Flea collars or tags are used extensively. If they are fresh when applied, they remain effective for several months. In areas with high temperatures and low humidity, these remedies seem to be more toxic to the pet. The flea collar works by enveloping the pet in a cloud of insecticidal vapor. It is more effective on a sedentary pet, since with an active pet the "cloud" may dissipate and thus be ineffective. Flea collars that are too tight, moistened a lot, or used in other incorrect ways may produce a local skin reaction or even a severe generalized effect. This is especially true with cats. Apply the fresh collar with due attention to the manufacturer's instructions. Remove it at the first sign of irritation.

Simultaneous treatment of the premises is mandatory for good flea control. If infestation is severe, hire a commercial exterminator. Thoroughly vacuum rugs, floors, and especially those areas where your pet sleeps or spends a lot of time, to help remove flea eggs and larvae. Then burn the vacuumed dust. Flea bombs or foggers may be useful if repeated often, but residual sprays or dusts applied to cracks in the floor and cool cement flooring are more effective. The yellow vaponna fly strips are also effective in flea control. Hang one in the area of the room most frequented by the pet or—ideally—fix part of a strip to the inside roof of a doghouse and place the rest of the strip *under* the floor of the doghouse. This keeps the pet's sleeping quarters treated constantly with insecticidal vapor—with low toxic potentials, since the pet will only be there periodically. The pet gets a treatment every time it takes a nap. Oral medications for control of fleas on your pet have not been highly effective.

LICE

Lice are wingless insects with flattened bodies. They spend their entire life cycle on the animal and are easily eliminated. They can exist only a few days away from a host. There are two types of lice: biting and sucking. Lice are spread by direct contact or by combs and brushes that are used on several animals. Lice cause intense itching and may cause such distress that the pet becomes irritable and restless. The life cycle of lice is one to three weeks. The eggs, or nits, are white particles firmly attached to the hair. Treat with dusts, sprays, or dips (as for fleas) and repeat the treatment 2 or 3 times at 7- to 14-day intervals. Simultaneously treat all animals in contact with one another.

TICKS

Ticks are large, pea-sized, insectlike creatures, which are usually found attached to the skin of your pet. They may be present on any part of the body but are most abundant around the head and toes. Ticks have several stages in their life cycle. They usually feed on other hosts, such as small rodents or wild animals, during part of the cycle. Although there are both hard and soft ticks, the former are a greater problem for pet animals. Although the actual tick bite is rarely serious and causes no pain, these parasites may transmit several serious infectious diseases, so their control is important. Do *not* try to remove the tick by using a lighted cigarette. If there are only a few ticks, soak them with rubbing alcohol (or even gin). The tick soon becomes stupefied and either backs out of the skin or can be plucked off easily with a tweezer. In the latter case, grasp the tick as close to the skin as possible and pull steadily (it is desirable to remove the head). Then place the tick in a jar of alcohol for a few minutes and either burn it or flush it down the toilet.

Some ticks may invade the kennel or your home, where they live in cracks between floorboards and between the floors and walls. Control in these cases is difficult, and you should hire a commercial exterminator. Ticks are especially troublesome in wooded areas near coastal beaches and in rural mountain areas. They have definite seasons, and control of the problem outside your home is virtually impossible. Periodic dusting, spraying, or continuous use of flea and tick collars may be of some help.

MANGE MITES

These tiny insectlike creatures are barely visible with the naked eye. Four types of mange are briefly discussed here: demodectic mange, sarcoptic mange, ear mange, and cheyletiella, or "walking dandruff." Mange mites all have direct life cycles and spend their entire life on the host animal. They will live only a few days away from the host. Demodectic mange is not contagious, but all the other forms are. Diagnosis in all cases is made by microscopic examination of a skin scraping.

DEMODECTIC MANGE

This type of mange tends to run in families and is acquired from the mother at birth (the only time it may be transmitted). If you discover that your new puppy has demodectic mange, consider taking it back to the seller for a refund or a replacement. A pet may have a mild form of demodectic mange, which does not itch but results in hair loss from areas around the face and legs. Most such cases are easy to treat; many heal spontaneously at the time of sexual maturity. A second and more severe form of the disease is complicated by serious bacterial skin infections. The skin may be red and ooze pus. Treatment is long and expensive—definitely a problem for your veterinarian to solve.

SARCOPTIC MANGE

Sarcoptic mange causes intense itching. It is highly contagious, and an animal may even transmit it to man. In people, however, the mites only live for a few days unless reinfection occurs. In cats the disease is called head mange and is characterized by crusted, hairless lesions around the ears, face, elbows, and tail. In dogs the lesions are hairless, and the pet usually scratches them raw. Here, too, the ears, face, elbows, and legs are most commonly affected. Special insecticidal solutions are necessary for both types, and it is wise to seek veterinary advice for diagnosis and initial treatment. Apply treatment thoroughly to all parts of all animals in contact with one another. Repeat the treatment weekly for at least four weeks. It is not necessary to treat the premises more than once.

EAR MANGE

Ear mange affects both dogs and cats and is also contagious. It causes itching, shaking of the head, and secondary infection of the ear canals. The mites spend most of their time in the ears, so concentrate treatment there. However, some of these mites may travel to other parts of the body, so also treat the entire body with flea sprays or dusts. Mild infection may persist for months. Try to eliminate the problem by vigorous and thorough treatment in its early stages.

"WALKING DANDRUFF"

This is a mild skin problem caused by large white mites that live on the surface of the skin. The mites resemble flakes of dandruff, and if you look closely or use a magnifying lens, you can see them move. They are commonly found on puppies kept in crowded conditions (this mange is highly contagious and can be transmitted to man). The mites cause the "dandruff" along the top of the back and moderate itching. These mites affect cats and dogs; however, with cats the condition is milder and there is less itching.

To treat, apply the powders and sprays used to control fleas 2 or 3 times weekly for 2 or 3 weeks.

35.

Vaccinations

Immunization procedures for cats and dogs have benefited immeasurably in the last decade from the development of new vaccines and methods of application. Veterinarians now routinely expect vaccines to be almost perfectly effective. This, of course, is impossible, but many diseases that were the bane of our pets just a few years ago are rare today. This is especially true among pets that are properly vaccinated. Fresh, potent vaccines administered in the proper way at the proper time are undoubtedly the greatest bargain in veterinary medicine today. Unfortunately, unvaccinated animals, especially strays, pose a constant threat to our pets. It is imperative that each pet be kept current in its vaccinations against the preventable diseases.

The recommended time schedules for vaccinating dogs and cats can be confusing, but they really do make sense. When puppies or kittens are born, they have no immune protection to infectious diseases, but when the young suckle for the first time, during their first day of life, this changes. The mother's first milk (colostrum) contains protective antibodies against any of the infections to which *she* is immune. For this reason, it is most important that newborn puppies and kittens receive that first milk. Depending on the degree of the mother's immunity, the young will have a temporary (passive) protection that lasts from a few weeks to as long as four months. By testing the mother's blood, your veterinarian can tell you more precisely when to vaccinate. If you cannot have the test, remember that most puppies and kittens lose their maternal protection by 9 or 10 weeks of age. It is important to know this time because the mother's antibodies not only protect the young from disease but interfere with the beneficial action of the vaccines. There is no absolute schedule, and one must gamble somewhat on when to start immunizations.

The general recommendations (modified in some areas according to local problems) are:

1. Be sure the young receive their mother's milk the first day of life.

2. Keep the young isolated from other animals or possible disease sources—especially between 3 and 8 or 9 weeks of age.

3. Present the litter to your veterinarian for immunization at 8 or 9 weeks of age. Usually several injections will be needed at intervals of several weeks.

Vaccinations for Dogs

It is now recommended that dogs be protected against
Rabies
Distemper
Canine hepatitis
Leptospirosis (two types)
Infectious bronchitis (kennel cough)

Several of the above are combined in a single injection. All except rabies can be started at 2 months of age and completed at 4 months of age. Annual boosters are strongly recommended. In some areas leptospirosis vaccine may be omitted; in other areas it must be repeated at less than a one-year interval.

Rabies vaccine should not be given to puppies before they are 4 months old. It must be repeated at three-year intervals and is usually mandated as a public-health measure. The dog must have a current rabies vaccination before it can be licensed. It is necessary to vaccinate a dog for rabies before it can be shipped across state lines.

Vaccinations for Cats

It is now recommended that cats be protected against
Rabies
Panleukopenia (feline distemper)
Feline upper-respiratory disease (two viral diseases)

Some of these vaccines are combined in a single injection. One type of vaccine must be given intramuscularly, while another is given by droplets placed in the eye and the nostril. Your veterinarian will have a preference about which will be best for your pet. Vaccination usually starts at 8 weeks of age and should be completed by 16 weeks. Annual boosters are strongly recommended.

Rabies vaccine cannot be given to kittens before 4 months of age. It must be repeated annually. If a cat is to be kept as a house pet exclusively and never allowed outdoors, you may consider omitting the rabies vaccination. Consult your veterinarian. A cat being shipped across state lines must have a current rabies vaccination.

36.

Housebreaking a Pet

Dogs

Dogs must be housebroken, and you can accomplish this easily if everyone in the household concentrates on the problem for a short, intensive training period. A young puppy usually needs to urinate every 2 to 3 hours during the day. Watch closely as this time interval approaches. When the puppy starts sniffing and looking around the floor, hustle it to the newspaper toilet area indoors or to the selected toilet area outside. Reward performance in the proper place with praise and other methods of positive reinforcement.

A puppy is naturally clean and will try to avoid messing its sleeping quarters. Use this trait to advantage by allowing the puppy to relieve itself late in the evening and then confining it in its bed area for the night. The area of confinement should be small: just large enough so the puppy can be comfortable—and no larger. An ideal method is to tie the puppy with a collar and short leash, giving it just enough room to turn around in its bed. Then, early in the morning, take the puppy to the designated toilet area. Prompt urination will result. Again give positive reinforcement. A few days of this type of training is usually enough to establish the routine that leads to satisfactory housebreaking. However, carelessness or neglect on the owner's part will rapidly reverse the early progress. As the puppy matures, you can extend the intervals between trips to the toilet area, but do not confine even mature, well-trained dogs for more than 8 to 12 hours, else they, too, may err.

Dogs usually have the urge to pass stool 15 to 30 minutes after eating, so time exercise romps or visits to the toilet area according to this schedule, too. Animals are creatures of habit, and we should do everything we can to reinforce *good* habits. That is training.

If you expect your dog to use an outdoor site for the toilet area, you must set up a rigid schedule. Always go out the same door; go to the selected place each time and allow the dog to sniff around and investigate the area; leave urine and some stool in place to remind your pet, by sight and smell, of why it is there. This works well in an indoor area, too; leave a piece of the soiled paper on top of the new paper in the designated toilet area.

Persistence and consistency result in rapid training. Keep at it—and good luck!

Cats

Cats are naturally clean and do not need special toilet training. They should have either a special, secluded litter box as a toilet area or frequent access to the out-of-doors. A cat will bury its urine and feces and clean itself afterward; so it makes an ideal apartment pet. If your cat is constantly indoors, you can keep the litter box odor-free and sanitary by locating it in an out-of-the-way place and cleaning it frequently. Remove the feces with a coarse strainer or spoon and flush them down the toilet. Replace the entire litter weekly or as needed. Fresh litter can be made up of shredded newspapers or, better yet, one of the dustfree clay-particle products sold commercially. Avoid those products that are dusty, as they may cause respiratory problems.

When a cat that has been fastidious about its toilet habits suddenly forgets its training, this may be due to organic disease involving the urinary or digestive tract (diarrhea). However, a cat will sometimes develop a neurosis or anxiety state that causes it to fail to bury its stool, to spray urine on the rugs and furniture, or to overeat and become obese. The cat's personality may change, too. These problems may be caused by the addition of a new cat to the neighborhood or to the household or even a new baby in the family. Your pet then feels displaced in the pecking order of its society. Loss of a favorite plaything, a new sleeping box or food dish, or special changes in daily routine may also cause the neurosis. Try to pinpoint the exact time the behavioral change started and determine what factors might have caused it. Then attempt to correct these factors or compensate for them. Sometimes the remedy is obvious, and sometimes it is impossible. Your veterinarian may be able to assist you in understanding cat psychology; but in any case, have your pet examined to eliminate organic disease as a possible cause.

37.

Removing Urine
from Rugs and Furniture

When removing urine, you will achieve best results if you act promptly. Use the following:

1. Blot up the urine with paper towels.
2. Scrub the area several times with white vinegar, blotting it dry each time. Stroke inward to localize the stain.
3. Cover the area with cornstarch or baking soda (dry powder) and leave for 4 hours, until the urine is absorbed.
4. Vacuum up the powder thoroughly.

Commercial products designed to remove urine odor and stain are available for home use and have been used with variable success. Sometimes it is necessary to employ a commercial rug or upholstery cleaner as a last resort.

It is essential that the odor and stain be removed. When the odor of urine or bowel movements remains in an area, it reminds a pet of the need to relieve itself. In fact, an animal "marks" its toilet areas this way. This habit can be used to advantage in successfully housebreaking a pet (see page 230).

To prevent accidents, *don't* allow odor hints to remain in forbidden areas. Clean up accidents promptly and thoroughly.

To help in housebreaking, *do* leave odor hints on newspapers or in desired toilet areas outdoors—at least until your pet forms correct habits (see page 230).

Reasons for Urine Accidents

1. Keeping the pet confined for too long a period of time (4 to 8 hours is the maximum interval for most normal pets).
2. Litter box or newspaper areas not available to the pet.
3. Disease condition.
    a. Urinary infections, bladder stones, or tumors.
    b. Abnormally high water intake.
4. Anxiety. Cats, particularly, may spray urine on furniture or lose housebreaking when they become neurotic or displaced in the pecking order of their territorial environment. Nervous, anxious, or shy dogs may squat or roll on their backs and urinate when approached aggressively by other dogs or by people—especially strangers.

38.

Motion Sickness

Definition

Motion sickness is nausea and vomiting produced by riding in cars, airplanes, boats, and other moving vehicles.

Causes

Motion sickness is caused by a continuous stimulation of the balance centers in the inner ear. This rarely seems to bother young puppies and kittens or older dogs and cats. The majority of problems occur in immature, or young-adult pets. Cats are usually more tolerant of motion than dogs.

When an animal becomes upset during travel it *may* have true motion sickness; but many pets are really only showing the effects of nervousness, excitement, or fear of the car, the car's odors, or of an unpleasant experience during the trip.

Signs and Symptoms

1. There are varying degrees of illness. Usually a pet becomes quiet and depressed; it may pant, retch, and salivate profusely. Vomiting and diarrhea may develop in advanced cases. The illness is never fatal, and recovery occurs within a few minutes after motion ceases.

2. An animal may become emotionally upset by travel but is still thought to have motion sickness. These patients may pace, breathe rapidly, act afraid, and often have enlarged pupils and

look "bug-eyed." They may cry, scratch at the vehicle doors, and jump around excessively. Unless restrained, they are very distracting to the other occupants and may be dangerous to the operator of the car.

FIRST AID FOR MOTION SICKNESS

1. Stop the motion and let the animal rest. Recovery is rapid.

2. Use newspapers or cloths to clean up messes of saliva, vomited material, or stool.

Prevention

1. Train your pet to travel well by taking it on short trips—especially those that end in pleasant experiences. Placing an animal in a car for a short while, feeding it in the car, traveling to a local market or for a romp in the country, all represent positive training.

2. *Always* transport a cat in a small comfortable cat carrier. The type with wire ends for ventilation and a blanket pad on the bottom for comfort is ideal. It may be wise to confine the cat to the carrier for several nights at home so it becomes used to the carrier as a shelter and haven. Leave the door of the carrier open at home so the cat can seek it out as a safe, cavelike retreat. Cats that are allowed loose in automobiles may bolt out the door when you stop and become hopelessly lost many miles from home. An unnecessary tragedy!

3. Observe the following rules for almost all traveling pets.
   a. Do not feed the animal for 6 hours before departure.
   b. Restrict water for 12 hours before departure and remove it completely for the last hour.
   c. Exercise just before departure to allow bowel and urine elimination.
   d. Do not feed or give water to your pet en route unless the trip will be more than 12 to 18 hours. (Dogs that do not

develop motion sickness can be given small amounts of water at rest stops.)

e. Apply a collar and leash so that dogs can be exercised at rest stops every 2 to 4 hours.

f. Provide good ventilation but do not allow the pet to ride in the rear of an open truck or to put its head out a window.

4. If necessary, use preventive medication for motion sickness. Your veterinarian can provide you with tranquilizers, antihistamines, or combination drugs, which are often effective in controlling motion and excitement problems. Each pet has specific problems, and each may react better to one drug or combination than to another. It may take trial and error to find the best medication for your pet.

Meclizine HC1 (Bonine) is a nonprescription drug that is often helpful. You can procure it from veterinarians or from drugstores. Administer Bonine orally one hour before departure. Give very small (toy) dogs 12.5 mg., medium-sized dogs (25 to 50 lbs.) 25 mg., and large dogs (over 50 lbs.) 50 mg. in a like manner. The effect lasts at least 12 hours.

If these regimes do not work, carefully observe your pet's actions during travel, report them to your veterinarian, and have him prescribe special medications tailored to your pet's needs.

39.

Vomiting

Definition

Vomiting is a centrally controlled, reflex act during which the stomach contracts and ejects its contents through the mouth.

Causes

Dogs and cats can vomit more easily than many other species; some people believe they can do this voluntarily. Vomiting is an important protective mechanism because it allows pets to empty their stomachs of toxic, spoiled, or irritating substances easily and quickly. You may even want to encourage vomiting if your pet has recently ingested such substances. Many dogs and cats eat grass—in fact some individuals almost "graze," they eat so much. The grass may stimulate vomiting, but it is not a serious problem.

Food that is ejected from the mouth may be vomited from the stomach or it may be regurgitated—that is, brought up from storage in a dilated esophagus. In this latter case, the food looks as if it has just been eaten, but it is sausage-shaped and covered with foam.

Some animals that cough and bring up fluids from the lungs and throat are mistakenly thought to be vomiting. These "coughs" involve much snorting and gagging; the dog puts its head down, hacks, and spits out a small amount of mucus or sticky fluid.

Be sure you are treating *vomiting*—not regurgitation or a productive cough.

Vomiting can be caused by many disorders. Dietary change, hot or cold food, overeating, indigestion, poisons, drugs, intestinal or gastric foreign bodies, infectious diseases (cat distemper, hepatitis), throat infection, kidney failure, ear problems, and motion sickness are just a few examples.

Vomiting can be a simple problem and easily solved; but if it persists, it can be most serious. It is very stressful and tiring, and it results in the loss of water, minerals, and nutrients, which the animal needs.

The procedures listed below are for simple vomiting, when the patient acts quite alert in other respects.

FIRST AID FOR VOMITING

1. Remove or correct the cause if possible.

2. Withhold all food and water for 24 hours (medications excepted).

3. If the pet is very thirsty, give water in very small amounts frequently. Give only 1 or 2 teaspoonsful each time. Large amounts of water may actually increase the vomiting.

4. Give milk of bismuth or Pepto-Bismol frequently, as indicated in the dosage schedule on page 252.

5. Confine your pet, so it is warm, comfortable, and resting.

6. If vomiting has ceased, start feeding small amounts of broth, cooked egg, or *boiled* hamburger (with the fat poured off). Repeat the feeding every 2 to 4 hours, and if the response is good, gradually return to regular feeding in 1 to 2 days.

40.

Hairballs

All cats lick themselves frequently as a method of grooming and cleaning. A cat's tongue has many fine barbs, which tend to force the cat to swallow material caught in the mouth instead of spitting it out. A long-haired cat will swallow large amounts of hair as a result of licking. This may wad up into a dense, feltlike mass in the stomach. The hairball is a space-occupying mass, so the cat feels full, is not hungry, and may not eat normally. As a result, it may lose weight. Eventually, some of the hair will be passed in the stool or brought up by vomiting. In rare cases, the hair may be irritating and form a large mass that requires veterinary treatment.

Hairballs can usually be prevented by frequent and thorough combing and brushing to remove loose hair or by oral treatment with oil. Periodically (once or twice a month) give your cat *mineral oil*. It will soak into the mass of hair, compress it, and allow it to be passed in the stool. Add about 1 teaspoon of mineral oil to the cat's food daily for 3 days. As an alternative, place a large glob of *white* petroleum jelly on the cat's nose. The cat will lick it off and swallow it, and in the warm stomach, it will turn to mineral oil. After the 3 days of oil treatment, give a mild laxative—1 to 2 teaspoons of milk of magnesia—to hasten the hair on its way through the intestines.

Never "dose" mineral oil by forcing it into the cat. It may be inhaled and cause pneumonia. Do not give oil more frequently than recommended here. To do so prevents absorption of many nutrients and vitamins. And since mineral oil is not digested or absorbed, excess amounts leak out of the cat's anus and stain your furniture.

41.

Diarrhea and Flatulence (Gas)

Diarrhea

Diarrhea is the frequent passage of unformed stools. They are often liquid, have a foul odor, and may be passed frequently and with urgency.

CAUSES

1. Excessive fat, milk, or uncooked starch.
2. Cold food.
3. Sudden dietary changes.
4. Spoiled food or garbage.
5. Internal parasites (worms).
6. Allergies to specific foods (milk, wheat, or seafoods).
7. Poisons of various kinds.
8. Continual stress and anxiety.

More serious causes of diarrhea include infections, systemic diseases, digestive or absorption disorders, and tumors.

Seek veterinary care for long-standing diarrheas and those that result in weight loss and are unresponsive to treatment.

FIRST AID FOR DIARRHEA

1. Try to determine if there has been a diet change or other modification of the usual routine which could explain the diarrhea. Remove or correct the cause if possible.

2. Withhold all food for 24 hours. Allow access to plain water.

3. Give large, frequent doses of kaolin and pectin, as directed in the appendix section under drug dosages (page 252). Do not skimp on the medication! Continue medication for at least 3 days.

4. After 24 hours, start feeding fresh beef boiled in salted water. Gradually add cooked eggs, toast, and finally, small amounts of dry dog food to the meat and broth. Gradually return the animal to regular feeding.

5. If the diarrhea persists or if blood or mucus is present, collect a fresh typical stool sample and take it with your pet to your veterinarian.

Flatulence (Gas)

This annoying problem results from gulping food (and thus swallowing air), from eating spicy or starchy foods, or from a diet high in meat or eggs. It may be difficult to control, but experimenting with the diet and feeding charcoal tablets after meals may help relieve the problem.

42.

Constipation

Definition

Constipation is the difficult and infrequent passage of stools.

Causes and Prevention

Constipation may be caused when an animal eats large amounts of bone; dry, indigestible food; bedding, wood, or other foreign material. This condition is aggravated if there is an obstruction in the pelvic area (such as a fracture, tumor, or hernia) also blocking the passage of stools. Many animals become more easily constipated as they grow older because, as they receive less exercise, their muscle tone decreases.

A constipated animal will strain unsuccessfully to pass feces, appear listless, and lose its appetite.

Caution: A cat with a urinary obstruction will sit in its litter box and strain, as if it were constipated. Be careful to diagnose the situation correctly, as a urinary obstruction is an emergency and requires immediate veterinary care (see pages 115–116).

You can help prevent constipation by feeding your pet food that is well-soaked in water to make it soft and moist. Milk and liver tend to have a laxative effect; give them several times a week with your pet's regular diet. Brewer's yeast and vitamin B complex are also useful in preventing constipation. *Do not* give your pet laxatives on a regular basis, as they may be habit forming. Also, do not give your pet mineral oil routinely, as it may prevent the absorption of many nutrients, and, if inhaled, may produce a serious lung condition. Use laxatives only when necessary and only for a short period of time.

FIRST AID FOR CONSTIPATION

MILD CONSTIPATION

1. Give your pet equal parts of milk of magnesia and mineral oil (see page 253).

2. As an alternative, give your dog or cat the mineral oil treatment for cats with hairballs (see page 240).

SEVERE CONSTIPATION

1. Give an enema (see pages 194–197).

2. If relief does not occur, consult your veterinarian.

43.

Pedicures:
Ingrown and Bleeding Toenails

Dogs

Old dogs or dogs that do not exercise much may develop long toenails. On occasion the nails will curl around and grow back into the skin of the foot pad. This is especially true of dewclaws—the small toes (on the side of the legs) that do not contact the ground.

It is easy to keep your dog's nails trimmed. Purchase special nail-clippers for that purpose. Cut the nails at an angle perpendicular to the long axis of the nail and about ¼ inch outside the pink mark, which identifies the blood supply. (See Figure 50, page 246.) Train your dog as a puppy to accept combing, ear-cleaning, and nail-trimming, and the tasks will be easy. If you accidentally cut the nail too short, so it bleeds, do not panic. It may hurt, but you can easily control the bleeding. Draw the bleeding nail across a bar of softened soap. The soap will "pack" into the end of the nail and effectively control the hemorrhage.

If a dewclaw nail has grown into the soft tissue of the leg, cut the nail at the proper place and extract the embedded tip of the nail. Treat the small puncture as you would any infected wound —cleanse and apply antibacterial dressings (see pages 29 and 255). The wound will heal rapidly, and your pet will be grateful for the relief you have provided.

Broken toenails usually result when long nails are caught in rugs or between stones. Since the break is often not complete and the nail hangs on by a small piece of tissue, it is constantly moving and is very painful. Grasp the broken nail segment, and with a hard,

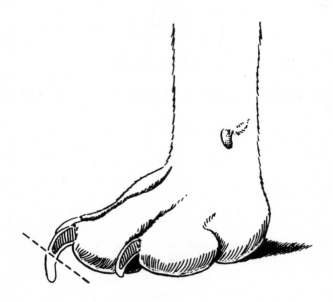

FIGURE 50. *A pedicure.* Trim the nail at the angle and at the location of the dotted line. The shaded area of the nail indicates the "pink" blood supply.

twisting motion, pull the broken piece off. You can also cut it with clippers, but this produces hemorrhaging. Stop bleeding by the soap method described above.

Cats

Cats keep their nails sharp by honing them on carpets, furniture, or tree trunks. If you clip their nails, they will soon be sharp again. Having the nails of the front feet surgically removed is a good idea—especially for indoor cats. They are not really handicapped and, when outdoors, they can still climb trees quite well. Indoors, they can't scratch furniture or people.

44.

Porcupine Quills

Porcupines are common in rural woodlands, especially in the northern parts of the United States and in Canada. Porcupines and hedgehogs have tough, spinelike quills of varying lengths, which completely cover their bodies except for the faces, feet, and soft underbellies. When attacked, they roll up in a ball and use their quills as excellent protection from marauding dogs or wild predators. A porcupine cannot "throw" quills, but if an animal bites the quills, they may loosen and stick in the paws or mouth of the attacker. Each quill has many tiny barbules on the end; so once they pierce the skin or mucous lining of the mouth, they are difficult to remove.

Dogs are the worst offenders. They are usually curious about porcupines and may paw or sniff them. If the dog is lucky, it is speared by only a few quills and learns never to bother another "porky." However, some dogs become aggressive, and in spite of the pain, bite the procupine repeatedly and even shake it viciously. These dogs can be pierced by literally hundreds of quills. Treatment to remove quills is painful unless anesthesia is used. If your dog has many quills imbedded in its skin, take it to a veterinary hospital for anesthesia and careful, humane removal. Some quills penetrate deeply under the skin or in the throat and may require surgical removal. If left in place, these quills tend to migrate and may cause complications. If only a few quills are present, the pain of leaving them and the pain of removal may be equal. If professional aid is not available, the owner should remove them.

FIRST AID FOR PORCUPINE QUILLS

1. Muzzle and restrain the dog.

2. Use a surgical hemostat, a needle-nosed pliers, or even ordinary pliers if nothing better is at hand.

3. Grasp each quill firmly near the skin and remove it with a firm "twitch," pulling in the exact direction of the long axis of the quill. Do not pull at an angle—or the quill may break. The tiny barbules hold the quills very firmly in place.

4. Since the quills may introduce infection, consult your veterinarian about possible antibiotic therapy.

5. Observe your pet carefully for about a week. Look for signs of infection, abscess formation, or quills working their way out of deep locations in the tissues.

6. Keep your pet away from the wooded areas frequented by porcupines and keep it confined at night—the time when most dog-and-porcupine confrontations seem to take place.

APPENDIXES

APPENDIX 1

Drug Dosages

Used properly, drugs help alleviate pain, control disease, and promote healing.

However, nature is the ultimate healer—medical measures are only aids. If we interfere with nature's methods, we may harm the patient, not help it.

Even the most innocuous substances, such as salt, can be harmful and even lethal if given in excess amounts.

Medication dosages for animal patients present special problems because there is no standard-sized animal. Dogs come in all sizes—from a 3-pound toy poodle puppy to a 140-pound Great Dane. Thus, dosages cannot be measured in units per patient, as they are for man.

It is imperative that you weigh your pet (especially if it is a dog) so you can better estimate the dosage of medication it needs. Cats usually vary less in weight; so feline doses are relatively standard.

If there is a question in your mind about dosage, use a low dose, or better yet withhold the medication and get specific veterinary advice. The following list includes a variety of medications that are relatively safe but effective for a number of common disorders, as well as indications for their use. Use these drugs either orally or externally (topically), as indicated.

Indications and Dosage

ORAL MEDICATIONS

Aspirin: helps reduce fever and relieve muscle and joint pain. Give with food, as it may upset the stomach.

> DOGS: 0.1 to 2.0 gms. every 12 hours.
> CATS: Do not use.

Bismuth or Pepto-Bismol: coats the stomach and is useful for the control of vomiting and diarrhea. Give frequently.

    DOGS: 1 tsp. per 20 lbs. of dog every 4 hours.

    CATS: ½ tsp. every 4 hours.

Brewer's yeast: a source of multiple B vitamins. It has an appealing flavor for dogs and cats.

    DOG: 0.1 gm. per lb. of dog once daily.

    CATS: Same.

Charcoal: absorbs toxic materials and thus prevents their absorption into the body. Is also an antiflatulence (gas) product. A very safe drug.

    DOGS: 2 heaping Tbsp. in 4 ounces of water per 30 lbs. of dog once, *or* 6 tablets per 30 lbs. of dog.

    CATS: 1 heaping tsp. in 1 ounce water once *or* 1 crushed tablet.

Cod-liver oil: a source of vitamin A and D. Do not give large doses or administer for long periods of time.

    DOGS: 1 tsp. per 20 lbs. of dog once daily.

    CATS: ¼ tsp. once daily.

Cough medicine: an expectorant mixture for short-term use in respiratory infections or coughing.

    DOGS: Guaifinesin, ½ to 1 tsp. every 4 hours.

    CATS: Guaifinesin, ¼ tsp. every 4 hours.

Hydrogen peroxide: a safe medication given by mouth to induce vomiting. Usually acts within 5 to 10 minutes.

    DOGS: 3% solution, 1 to 2 tsp. every 15 minutes until vomiting occurs.

    CATS: 3% solution, 1 tsp. every 15 minutes until vomiting occurs.

Kaolin-pectin solution (Kaopectate): a coating and binding material for use in diarrhea and certain poisonings. Give often and in full dosage, as it is very safe and underdosage decreases its value.

    DOGS: 1 tsp. per 5 lbs. of dog every 2 to 6 hours.

    CATS: Same.

Meclizine (Bonine): useful for motion sickness. Lasts 12 hours. It either works very well or is ineffective on an individual basis. Give

1 hour before traveling. Do not feed the animal before or during the trip.

DOGS: 25 mg. once daily. Dogs over 50 lbs., 50 mg. once daily.

CATS: 12.5 mg. once daily.

D-L methionine (Pedameth): a natural food substance that increases acidity of the urine. It is often used in urinary infections.

DOGS: 0.2 to 1.0 gm. every 8 hours.

CATS: 0.2 gm. every 8 hours.

Milk of magnesia: an antacid and laxative. It is used for constipation, as an antacid, and to flush toxic materials from the intestinal tract by cathartic action.

DOGS: 1 tsp. per 5 lbs. of dog, up to maximum of 8 tsp., once.

CATS: 1 tsp. per 5 lbs. of cat, once.

Mineral oil: a lubricating material that is not digested or absorbed. It is a lubricant and laxative when given by mouth. It is best given with food (especially to cats where it is used to evacuate hairballs), because it is tasteless. If it is not given with food, it may run into the trachea and cause a lung reaction.

DOGS: 1 tsp. per 5 lbs. Single maximum dose 10 tsp. May be repeated in 12 hours.

CATS: ½ tsp. per 5 lbs. of cat. May be repeated in 12 hours.

Paregoric: an opium derivative that allays stomach cramps and diarrhea. Often combined with bismuth or kaolin-pectin mixture.

DOGS: ½ tsp. per 10 lbs. every 6 hours. Single maximum dose 1 tsp.

CATS: Do not use.

Sodium bicarbonate: an antacid to neutralize acid in the stomach or to alkalinize the urine.

DOGS: 25 mg. per lb. of dog every 8 hours.

CATS: Same.

Sodium dioctyl sulfosuccinate (Colace): a stool-softener that causes water to penetrate hard stool.

DOGS: 100 to 300 mg. every 12 hours.

CATS: 100 mg. every 12 hours.

Vitamin C: used to acidify the urine in treatment of urinary infections.
> DOGS: 100 to 500 mg. every 12 hours.
> CATS: 100 mg. every 12 hours.

TOPICAL APPLICATIONS

Aluminum acetate solution (Domeboro solution): a drying, astringent solution for insect bites and moist and irritated skin lesions.
> DOGS OR CATS: Add 1 packet *or* tablet to 1 cup tepid water and soak affected skin for 15 minutes 3 times daily.

Antibacterial ointments:
> *For the skin* (Neopolycin, Neosporin, Betadine ointment, Betadine solution): Neopolycin and Neosporin are antibiotic combinations for skin infections, abscesses, or wounds. Betadine ointment is a bland iodine ointment for similar uses. Betadine solution is an iodine liquid for cleansing the skin and wounds.
> *For the eyes* (Neopolycin, Neosporin): Available by prescription for eye infections.
>> DOGS AND CATS (FOR THE SKIN):
>> Neopolycin ⎱
>> Neosporin ⎰ Apply gently to affected areas 2 or 3 times daily.
>> Betadine
>> DOGS AND CATS (FOR THE EYES):
>> Neopolycin ⎱ By prescription only. Apply to surface of the
>> Neosporin ⎰ eyeball 4 times daily.

A and D ointment: a bland ointment containing vitamins A and D. Stimulates the healing of wounds and is soothing to irritated skin.
> DOGS AND CATS: Apply gently to irritated skin or minor wounds to stimulate healing.

BFI powder: an antiseptic and drying wound powder for minor cuts, scratches, and irritations.
> DOGS AND CATS: Apply to irritated areas of skin daily.

Chlorine solution (Clorox): a solution used for irrigating infected wounds or for application to bacterial (i.e., impetigo) or fungal (ringworm) diseases of the skin.
> DOGS AND CATS: ½ tsp. to 1 cup water. Soak affected skin for 15 minutes 3 times daily.

Limesulfur solution (Vlem-Dome): used for several types of mange, ringworm, and infections, and when itching is prominent.

DOGS AND CATS: 1 tsp. concentrate to 1 pint hot water. Soak affected skin once daily. Allow to dry without rinsing.

Nivea Creme: a mild skin cream to soften hard, dry skin and add moisture. It is soothing and lubricating.

DOGS AND CATS: Apply to dry or crusted skin 3 times daily.

Shampoo, Johnson's Baby: a bland cleansing shampoo. Rinse well. (Joy Liquid dishwashing detergent is excellent, too.)

DOGS AND CATS: Use as bland shampoo for ordinary cleansing. Rinse well and dry the coat.

Sodium bicarbonate solution: a neutralizing rinse for acid burns.

DOGS AND CATS: 1 Tbsp. to 1 cup water. Flush skin burns from acids. Rinse.

Vinegar: a neutralizing rinse for alkali burns.

DOGS AND CATS: Flush full strength on skin burns from lye or alkalies. Rinse.

RECTAL APPLICATION

Fleet enema: a prepackaged saline enema solution. Indicated in minor constipation.

DOGS: Inject 1 to 4 ounces into the rectum, using the special nozzle-tipped plastic bottle.

CATS: Do not use. (Soap and water is preferred.)

Useful Information About Small Pets

	HAMSTER	RABBIT	MOUSE	RAT	GERBIL	GUINEA PIG	DOG	CAT
Weight at birth	2 gm.	100 gm.	1.5 gm.	5.5 gm.	3 gm.	100 gm.	100–500 gm.	100 gm.
Puberty	(F)28–31 days (best to breed 70 days) (M) 45 days	4–9 months	35 days	56–60 days	(F) 3–5 months (M) 10–12 weeks	(F) 20–30 days (M) 70 days	7–12 months	5–8 months
Duration of estrus cycle*	4 days	15–16 days	4 days	4 days	4 days	16 days	21 days	14 days
Gestation	16 days	28–36 days	19–21 days	21–23 days	24 days	62–72 days	63 days	63 days
Separation of adults during parturition and weaning	Yes	Yes	No	No	No (mates for life)	No	Yes	Yes
Number per litter	4–10	7	10	8–10	1–12	1–4	1–14	1–6
Eyes open	15 days	10 days	11–14 days	14–17 days	16–20 days	Prior to birth	13–15 days	13–15 days
Wean at	25 days	42–56 days	21 days	21 days	21 days	14–21 days or 160 gm.	6–7 weeks	7–8 weeks
Postpartum estrus	Within 24 hours	14 days	Within 24–48 hours	Within 24–48 hours	Within 24–72 hours	Within 24 hours	4 months	Varies

Body temperature (°F)	97–101	101–103.2	96.4–100	99.5–100.6	100.8	100.4–102.5	100–103	100–103
Daily adult water consumption	8–12 ml./day	80 ml./kg. body weight	3–3.5 ml./day	20–30 ml./day	4 ml./day	10 ml./100 gm. body weight	30 ml./kg. body weight	50 ml./kg. body weight
Daily adult food consumption (varies with age and condition)	7–12 gm./day	100–150 gm./day	2.5–4 gm./day	20–40 gm./day	10–15 gm./day	30–35 gm./day	Varies	Varies
Diet	Commercial rat, mouse, or hamster chow supplemented with kale,† cabbage,† apples, milk	Commercial rabbit pellets, greens in moderation	Commercial mouse chow	Commercial rat or mouse chow	Commercial mouse or rat chow (lowest fat possible), sunflower seeds	Commercial guinea pig chow, good quality hay, kale, cabbage, fruits (cannot rely on vitamin C levels of commercial ration)	Commercial dog food —dry, moist, or soft-moist	Commercial cat food— dry, moist, or semi-moist
Room temperature (°F)	65–75	62–68	70–80	76–78	65–80	65–75	65	65
Humidity (percent)	50	50	50	50	less than 50	50	50	50

* All species listed (except the dog) are seasonal polyestrus.

† Better source of vitamin C than.lettuce.

Modified from S. M. Schuchman, "Individual Care and Treatment of Mice, Rabbits, Rats, Guinea Pigs, Hamsters, and Gerbils," *Current Veterinary Therapy*, VI (Philadelphia: W. B. Saunders Co., 1977), p. 728.

APPENDIX 3

Usual Adult
Resting Temperature, Pulse,
and Respiration

	DOGS	CATS
Rectal temperature (°F)	100–103	100–103
(°C)	38– 39	38– 39
Pulse rate per minute	80–140	110–180
Respiratory rate per minute	10– 30	20– 30

The figures in the above table may vary markedly from individual to individual. All values—especially the pulse and respiratory rates—may increase as a result of excitement. Small breeds, puppies, and kittens will have values higher than those shown above.

APPENDIX 4

63-Day Perpetual Gestation Table for Dogs and Cats

```
nception—Jan.  1 2 3 4 5  6  7  8  9 10 11 12 13 14 15 16 17 18 19 20 21 22 23 24 25 26 27                    28 29 30 31
e—Mar.         5 6 7 8 9 10 11 12 13 14 15 16 17 18 19 20 21 22 23 24 25 26 27 28 29 30 31           Apr.  1  2  3  4

nception—Feb.  1 2 3 4 5  6  7  8  9 10 11 12 13 14 15 16 17 18 19 20 21 22 23 24 25 26                          27 28
e—Apr.         5 6 7 8 9 10 11 12 13 14 15 16 17 18 19 20 21 22 23 24 25 26 27 28 29 30              May    1  2

nception—Mar.  1 2 3 4 5  6  7  8  9 10 11 12 13 14 15 16 17 18 19 20 21 22 23 24 25 26 27 28 29              30 31
e—May          3 4 5 6 7  8  9 10 11 12 13 14 15 16 17 18 19 20 21 22 23 24 25 26 27 28 29 30 31     June   1  2

nception—Apr.  1 2 3 4 5  6  7  8  9 10 11 12 13 14 15 16 17 18 19 20 21 22 23 24 25 26 27 28                 29 30
e—June         3 4 5 6 7  8  9 10 11 12 13 14 15 16 17 18 19 20 21 22 23 24 25 26 27 28 29 30        July   1  2

nception—May   1 2 3 4 5  6  7  8  9 10 11 12 13 14 15 16 17 18 19 20 21 22 23 24 25 26 27 28 29              30 31
e—July         3 4 5 6 7  8  9 10 11 12 13 14 15 16 17 18 19 20 21 22 23 24 25 26 27 28 29 30 31     Aug.   1  2

nception—June  1 2 3 4 5  6  7  8  9 10 11 12 13 14 15 16 17 18 19 20 21 22 23 24 25 26 27 28 29                 30
e—Aug.         3 4 5 6 7  8  9 10 11 12 13 14 15 16 17 18 19 20 21 22 23 24 25 26 27 28 29 30 31     Sept.     1

nception—July  1 2 3 4 5  6  7  8  9 10 11 12 13 14 15 16 17 18 19 20 21 22 23 24 25 26 27 28 29              30 31
e—Sept.        2 3 4 5 6  7  8  9 10 11 12 13 14 15 16 17 18 19 20 21 22 23 24 25 26 27 28 29 30     Oct.   1  2

nception—Aug.  1 2 3 4 5  6  7  8  9 10 11 12 13 14 15 16 17 18 19 20 21 22 23 24 25 26 27 28 29              30 31
e—Oct.         3 4 5 6 7  8  9 10 11 12 13 14 15 16 17 18 19 20 21 22 23 24 25 26 27 28 29 30 31     Nov.   1  2

conception—Sept. 1 2 3 4 5  6  7  8  9 10 11 12 13 14 15 16 17 18 19 20 21 22 23 24 25 26 27 28              29 30
e—Nov.         3 4 5 6 7  8  9 10 11 12 13 14 15 16 17 18 19 20 21 22 23 24 25 26 27 28 29 30        Dec.   1  2

nception—Oct.  1 2 3 4 5  6  7  8  9 10 11 12 13 14 15 16 17 18 19 20 21 22 23 24 25 26 27 28 29              30 31
e—Dec.         3 4 5 6 7  8  9 10 11 12 13 14 15 16 17 18 19 20 21 22 23 24 25 26 27 28 29 30 31     Jan.   1  2

nception—Nov.  1 2 3 4 5  6  7  8  9 10 11 12 13 14 15 16 17 18 19 20 21 22 23 24 25 26 27 28 29                 30
e—Jan.         3 4 5 6 7  8  9 10 11 12 13 14 15 16 17 18 19 20 21 22 23 24 25 26 27 28 29 30 31     Feb.      1

nception—Dec.  1 2 3 4 5  6  7  8  9 10 11 12 13 14 15 16 17 18 19 20 21 22 23 24 25 26 27                    28 29 30 31
e—Feb.         2 3 4 5 6  7  8  9 10 11 12 13 14 15 16 17 18 19 20 21 22 23 24 25 26 27 28           Mar.  1  2  3  4
```

From R. W. Kirk and S. I. Bistner, *Handbook of Veterinary Procedures and Emergency Treatment,* II (Philadelphia: W. B. Saunders Co., 1975), p. 622.

APPENDIX 5

Composition of Animal Milks

Common or Domesticated Animals

	% Solids	% OF SOLIDS Fat	Protein	Carbohydrates
Mouse (Muridae)	25.8	46.9	34.9	12.4
Rat (Muridae)	26.5	47.5	34.7	12.5
Guinea Pig (Caviidae)	17.9	30.6	47.8	16.4
Hamster (Cricetidae)	26.4	47.7	34.0	12.8
Rabbit (Leporidae)	30.5	34.2	51.0	6.4
Cat (Felidae)	18.2	25.0	42.2	26.1
Dog (Canidae)	24.0	44.1	33.2	15.8
Pig (Suidae)	20.0	36.6	33.0	24.8
Sheep (Bovidae)	20.5	41.9	27.9	26.3
Goat (Bovidae)	12.8	32.0	29.0	32.8
Cow (Bovidae)	11.9	29.9	25.6	38.7
Horse (Equidae)	10.9	14.4	20.2	56.6
Donkey (Equidae)	9.5	9.5	17.6	68.2

Figures for all species were obtained from literature and are subject to error. Data courtesy of Smith-Douglas Division, Borden Chemical, Borden, Inc., Norfolk, Virginia 23501.

Significant portions of these values were calculated from data published by: Jennes, R., and Eloan, R. E., "The Composition of Milks of Various Species—A Review" in *Dairy Sci. Abstr. 32* (10), pp. 599–612, Review Article No. 158.

APPENDIX 6

Substitutes for Maternal Milk

		% OF SOLIDS		
	% Solids	Fat	Protein	Carbohydrates
Esbilac® (powder) replaces bitch's milk	98.4	44.1	33.2	15.8
Liquid Esbilac® replaces bitch's milk	15.3	44.1	33.2	15.8
KMR® (Formerly Tabbi-Lac) replaces queen's milk	18.2	25.0	42.2	26.1
SPF-Lac® replaces sow's milk	15.2	36.6	33.0	24.8
Foal-Lac® (Powder) replaces mare's milk	94.9	14.4	20.2	56.6

These commercial products are manufactured by Pet-Vet Products, Borden Chemical, Borden, Inc., Norfolk, Virginia 23501.

Esbilac, KMR, SPF-Lac, and Foal-Lac are registered tradesmarks of Borden, Inc.

Estimated Nutrient Requirements of Adult Dogs and Cats

Amounts per Kilogram of Body Weight per Day for an Average-Sized Adult

	Dog	Cat
Energy (cal.)	65	90
Protein (gm.)*	2.1	3.8
Fat (gm.)	1.3	6.0
Carbohydrate (gm.)†	10.1	—
Minerals		
Calcium (mg.)	200.0	100
Phosphorus (mg.)	160.0	90
Iron (mg.)	1.3	1.6
Copper (mg.)	0.20	0.1
Cobalt (mg.)	0.06	0.05
Sodium Chloride (mg.)	330	500
Potassium (mg.)	220	50
Magnesium (mg.)	11	3
Manganese (mg.)	0.11	0.03
Zinc (mg.)	0.11	0.10
Iodine (mg.)	0.03	0.10
Vitamins		
Vitamin A (IU)	100	1000
D (IU)	6.6	25
E (mg.)	2.0	3.0
K (mg.)	0.03	—
B_{12} (mg.)	0.0007	—

* The protein levels stated assume a high biologic value (approximately 85 percent) for the protein used. If poorer quality protein is fed, higher levels of protein may be needed.

† Although no dietary requirement for carbohydrate has been determined, carbohydrate is often used to provide additional energy in commercial diets.

From F. A. Kallfelz, "Pediatric Nutrition," in *Current Veterinary Therapy* V (Philadelphia: W. B. Saunders Co., 1974), p. 111.

Amounts per Kilogram of Body Weight per Day for an Average-Sized Adult

	Dog	Cat
Folic acid (mg.)	0.004	—
Riboflavin (mg.)	0.04	0.07
Pyridoxine (mg.)	0.02	0.10
Pantothenic Acid	0.05	0.25
Niacin (mg.)	0.24	1.30
Choline (mg.)	33.00	33.00
Thiamine (mg.)	0.02	0.30
Inositol (mg.)	—	3.0
Biotin (mg.)	—	30

APPENDIX 8

Energy and Protein Requirements of Growing Dogs and Cats

	REQUIREMENT IN DOG		REQUIREMENT IN CAT	
Age (weeks)	Protein (gm./kg./day)	Energy (cal./kg./day)	Protein (gm./kg./day)	(cal./kg./day) Energy
0–1	15.9	140	19.9	300
1–2	15.4	150	17.9	280
2–3	15.3	190	22.5	265
3–4	15.3	200	—	250
Weaning	6.6	130	22.5	225
Half-grown	3.6	100	6.0	170
Adult	2.1	65	3.8	90

From F. A. Kallfelz, "Pediatric Nutrition," in *Current Veterinary Therapy* V (Philadelphia: W. B. Saunders Co., 1974), p. 112.

APPENDIX 9

Sources of
Additional Information

Guthrie, Esther L. *Home Book of Animal Care.* New York: Harper & Row, 1966. (Information about birds, insects, snakes, and unusual wild animals.)

Kirk, R. W., and Bistner, S. I. *Handbook of Veterinary Procedures and Emergency Treatment,* 2d ed. Philadelphia: W. B. Saunders Co., 1975.

Nutrient Requirements of Dogs. Publ. ISBN: 0-309-02043-3. Committee on Animal Nutrition, Agricultural Board, National Academy of Sciences, National Research Council (Washington, D.C., 1972).

Nutrient Requirements of Laboratory Animals, Number 10. Publ. ISBN 0-309-02028-X. 2d rev. ed. Subcommittee on Laboratory Animals, Committee on Animal Nutrition, Agricultural Board, National Academy of Sciences, National Research Council (Washington, D.C., 1972).

Pinniger, R. S., ed. *Jones' Animal Nursing.* 2d ed. London and New York: Pergamon Press, 1972.

APPENDIX 10

Abbreviations Used in This Book

°F. = Degrees Fahrenheit

°C. = Degrees Celsius

1″, 2″ = one inch, two inches

tsp. = teaspoon (or 5 ml.)

Tbsp. = Tablespoon (or 15 ml.)

ml. = milliliter (or 15 drops)

oz. = ounce (or 30 ml.)

gm. = gram

mg. = milligram ($\frac{1}{1000}$ gm.)

kg. = kilogram

lbs. = pounds

cal. = calories

IU = international units

TPR = Temperature, Pulse rate,
Respiratory rate of a patient.
Also called the vital signs.

Index

ABOUT THE AUTHOR

Robert W. Kirk, D.V.M., is Professor of Small Animal Medicine, Chairman of the Department of Small Animal Medicine and Surgery, and Director of the Small Animal Clinic, New York State College of Veterinary Medicine, Cornell University. He has been a practicing veterinarian for over thirty years and is an internationally recognized veterinary authority. In addition to being a teacher, clinician, and veterinary consultant, he has also raised English pointers and a variety of other pets.

Dr. Kirk lives with his wife in Ithaca, New York. He is the author of several standard texts for veterinarians.

NOTES

NOTES

NOTES